GASTROINTESTINAL EMERGENCIES

TONY CK THAM
Consultant Gastroenterologist, Ulster Hospital, Dundonald,
Belfast, Northern Ireland, UK

and

JOHN SA COLLINS
Consultant Gastroenterologist, Royal Victoria Hospital,
Belfast, Northern Ireland, UK

with contributions from

JOHN MOOREHEAD
Consultant Surgeon, Ulster Hospital, Dundonald, Belfast,
Northern Ireland, UK

PAUL NEILLY
Consultant Surgeon, Altnagelvin Area Hospital, Londonderry,
Northern Ireland, UK

BMJ
Books

First published in 2000
by BMJ Books, BMA House, Tavistock Square,
London WC1H 9JR

www.bmjbooks.com

British Library Cataloguing in Publication Data
A catalogue record for this book is available from the British Library

ISBN 0–7279–1485–5

Cover design by Egelnick & Webb, London
Typeset by J&L Composition Ltd., Filey, North Yorkshire
Printed and bound by J W Arrowsmith Ltd., Bristol

Contents

A colour plate section can be found between pages 52 and 53.

Dedicated to our families:
Katie, Jennifer, Alison, and Caroline Tham
Florence, Rachel, Gillian, and Katie Collins

Acknowledgements

We would like to thank the following people.

Mr John Moorehead, Consultant Surgeon, Ulster Hospital, Dundonald, Belfast for his comments on some of the chapters relating to the stomach, pancreas, gallbladder and biliary tree.

Dr Michael Hyland, Consultant Radiologist, Ulster Hospital, Dundonald, for providing the radiological illustrations and for his input into their interpretation.

Dr Richard Wright, Consultant Radiologist, Ulster Hospital, Dundonald, for providing some of the radiological illustrations.

The junior medical staff of the Ulster Hospital, Dundonald who provided valuable feedback for some of the chapters.

Part I
Approach to specific
presentations

1 Acute dysphagia

Definition

Dysphagia refers to the sensation of food being hindered in its normal passage from the mouth to the stomach. Patients with dysphagia most frequently complain that food "sticks" or "just won't go down".

Dysphagia can be divided into two types:

- oropharyngeal dysphagia, i.e. inability to initiate act of swallowing, striated muscle affected
- oesophageal dysphagia, i.e. disorders affecting the smooth muscle of the oesophagus.

Odynophagia is pain on swallowing.

Globus is the sensation of a lump, fullness, or tightness in the throat.

Differential diagnosis

Aetiology of *dysphagia* can be divided into oropharyngeal dysphagia and oesophageal dysphagia. Please see Tables 1.1 and 1.2.

Odynophagia typically results from oesophageal mucosal inflammation. Please see Table 1.3.

Globus may be caused by gastro-oesophageal reflux, a structural lesion in the pharynx, larynx or neck; hypertensive upper oesophageal sphincter, or psychological causes.

History and examination

Please see Figure 1.1 for a diagnostic algorithm.

3

Table 1.1 Aetiology of oropharyngeal dysphagia.

Neurological disorders
Cerebrovascular disease
Amyotrophic lateral sclerosis
Parkinson's disease
Multiple sclerosis
Bulbar poliomyelitis
Wilson's disease
Cranial nerve injury
Brainstem tumours

Striated muscle abnormalities
Polymyositis
Dermatomyositis
Muscular dystrophies
Myasthenia gravis

Structural lesions
Inflammatory, e.g. pharyngitis, abscess, TB, syphilis
Head and neck tumours
Congenital webs
Plummer–Vinson syndrome
Cervical osteophytes
Surgical resection of the oropharynx
Pharyngeal pouch (Zenker's diverticulum)
Cricopharyngeal bar

Metabolic abnormalities
Hypothyroidism
Hyperthyroidism
Steroid myopathy

Oropharyngeal dysphagia

- Associated phenomena include nasal regurgitation, coughing during swallowing, dysarthria, and nasal speech due to palate weakness.
- There may be presence of a speech disorder, cranial nerve deficits, limb weakness and changes in sleep pattern, e.g. snoring.
- Dysphagia is usually only part of the symptom complex in contrast to oesophageal dysphagia where the dysphagia is usually the prominent manifestation.
- Patients should have a careful neurological examination and evaluation of the pharynx and larynx, including direct laryngoscopy.

Table 1.2 Aetiology of oesophageal dysphagia.

Neuromuscular/dysmotility disorders
Achalasia
Scleroderma
Diffuse oesophageal spasm
Nutcracker oesophagus
Hypertensive lower oesophageal sphincter
Vigorous achalasia
Nonspecific oesophageal dysmotility
Chagas' disease
Other collagen disorders

Mechanical lesions, intrinsic
Peptic stricture
Carcinoma
Oesophageal webs
Oesophageal diverticula
Lower oesophageal (Schatzki's) ring
Benign tumours
Foreign bodies
Pemphigoid, pemphigus

Mechanical lesions, extrinsic
Bronchial carcinoma or mediastinal nodes
Vascular compression
Mediastinal abnormalities
Cervical osteoarthritis

Table 1.3 Aetiology of odynophagia.

Infectious oesophagitis
  Candida
  Herpes
  Cytomegalovirus

Pill induced oesophagitis

Reflux oesophagitis

Radiation oesophagitis

Caustic injury

Oesophageal motility disorder

Oesophageal cancer

Graft versus host disease

Oesophageal foreign body

Oesophageal dysphagia

Three important questions are crucial:

1 Is it worse with solids or liquids?
2 Is the dysphagia intermittent or progressive?

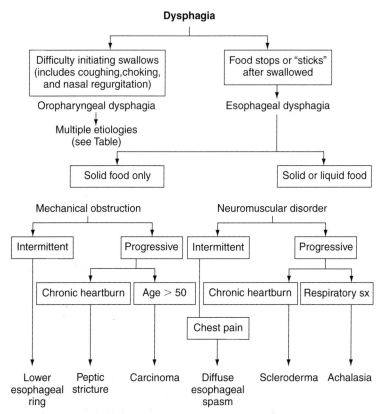

Figure 1.1 Diagnostic algorithm for the symptomatic assessment of the patient with dysphagia (From Castell DO. Approach to the patient with dysphagia. In: Yamada T, Alpers DH, Owyang C, Powell DW, Silverstein FE, eds. *Textbook of gastroenterology*. Philadelphia: Lippincott, 1995;638–48, with permission.)

3 Is there associated heartburn?

- The associated symptoms of chest pain and nocturnal coughing can suggest reflux or achalasia.
- Patients with mechanical obstruction usually have initial dysphagia for solids only and progress to dysphagia for liquids also. A relatively short history would suggest the presence of malignancy.
- Physical examination is usually not revealing. Presence of an abdominal mass and cervical glands should be looked for. In scleroderma other physical manifestations may be present.

Investigations

Barium swallow

- This is the preferred initial diagnostic test.
- If oropharyngeal dysphagia is suspected, videotaping a series of swallows provides imaging information that can be replayed at slower speed for careful diagnostic assessment.
- If oesophageal dysphagia is suspected, a solid bolus should be given to assess the ability to swallow solids.
- If the barium swallow suggests an obstructing lesion in the oesophagus, endoscopy should follow.
- If the radiographic findings suggest a motility disorder, an oesophageal motility study should be performed.

Endoscopy

- This should be performed in those with a normal barium swallow to rule out reflux oesophagitis or early oesophageal carcinoma which may be missed by a barium swallow. A prior barium swallow is not necessary in all cases. It allows biopsies to be performed and therapeutic dilatation of a stricture if present.

Oesophageal manometry

- This should be considered if both barium swallow and endoscopy are normal to evaluate motility disorders.
- It requires intubation of the oesophagus with a recording catheter which is connected to a physiograph. Pressure is recorded at predetermined recording orifices. Pressures at the lower oesophageal sphincter, oesophageal body and upper oesophageal sphincter are measured during wet swallows and bread swallows.

Management of dysphagia

The treatment of dysphagia depends on the aetiology.

Patients with *total dysphagia*, i.e. unable to swallow even small amounts of liquid or solid should be regarded as medical emergencies (see Figure 1.2).

Oropharyngeal dysphagia:

- Some patients have readily treatable disease, e.g. Parkinson's disease, myasthenia gravis, hypothyroidism.
- Those with dysphagia as a result of cerebrovascular accidents may benefit from being assessed by a speech therapist.

7

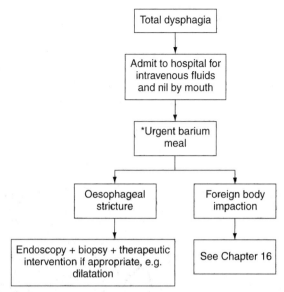

Figure 1.2 Management of total dysphagia (inability to even swallow liquids).
* or endoscopy

- Mechanical modifications and identifying which food consistencies are effectively swallowed without aspiration may help.
- If these measures fail, a PEG tube to facilitate enteral feeding may be considered.

Peptic stricture

- This may be dilated endoscopically using bougies or balloons. Some endoscopists routinely use fluoroscopy while others are more selective, using fluoroscopy only in complex strictures that would not allow passage of an endoscope.
- Almost all patients will get a symptomatic response.
- The risk of complications is low (see Chapter 18).
- All patients should be given maintenance proton pump inhibitors to reduce incidence of stricture recurrence.

Oesophageal carcinoma (Figure 1.3)

- Patients should have biopsies to confirm the diagnosis.
- The cancer should then be staged. The most accurate modality for staging is endoscopic ultrasound (accuracy in staging depth of invasion 87 –92% and regional lymph node status 80 – 88%).

A CT of the chest and abdomen is not as accurate (estimates from 39 to 100%) and has a tendency to understage. However if on CT there is definite evidence of invasion of vascular structures such as aorta or metastatic disease, this precludes curative resection. MRI has little advantage over CT.

- Surgery is the only hope for cure but only a few patients will be suitable for this. Contraindications to surgery include: invasion of vascular structures, metastatic disease, unfit patients with significant comorbid disease. There is no consensus that adjuvant radiation or chemotherapy should be used at present.

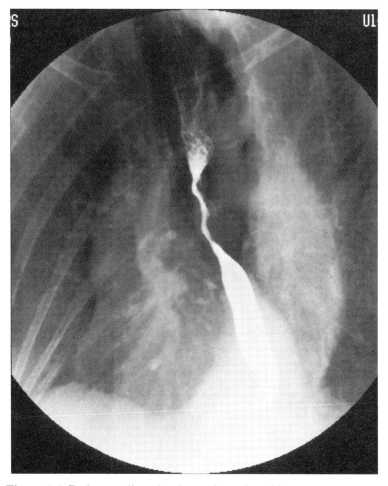

Figure 1.3 Barium swallow showing an irregular mid-oesophageal stricture with shouldering consistent with carcinoma.

- Options for palliation include oesophageal stent placement with metal self expanding stents, laser therapy, bipolar electrocoagulation therapy, photodynamic therapy, dilatation, radiotherapy, alcohol injection into the tumour, PEG tube placement. The best palliative modality should be individualised for the patient taking into account factors such as tumour morphology, anatomy, local expertise.

Achalasia

- Manometry is the preferred method to make the diagnosis. There is an absence of peristalsis in the body of the oesophagus (essential for diagnosis), incomplete relaxation of the lower oesophageal sphincter (residual pressure > 5 mm Hg), hypertensive lower oesophageal sphincter (> 45 mm Hg) and intraoesophageal pressure that is greater than intragastric pressure.
- Treatment options include surgical Heller's myotomy (response in 65–92%, long term complication of reflux in < 10%, mortality < 2%) or endoscopic pneumatic balloon dilatation (response in 32–98%, perforation in 1–13%, mortality rare).
- If the patient is unfit for these procedures, endoscopic injection of botulinum toxin into the lower oesophageal sphincter may produce short term benefit.

Further reading

1 American Society for Gastrointestinal Endoscopy. Esophageal dilation. Guidelines for clinical application. *Gastrointest Endosc* 1991;**32**:122.
2 Castell DO. Approach to the patient with dysphagia. In: Yamada T, Alpers DH, Owyang C, Powell DW, Silverstein FE, eds. *Textbook of gastroenterology*. Philadelphia: Lippincott, 1995;638-48.
3 Csendes A, Braghetto I, Henriquez A, Cortes C. Late results of prospective randomized study comparing forceful dilatation and oesophageomyotomy in patients with achalasia of the oesophagus. *Gut* 1989;**30**:299.
4 Knyrim K, Wagner HJ, Bethge N, Keymling M, Vakil N. A controlled trial of an expansile metal stent for palliation of esophageal obstruction due to inoperable cancer. *N Engl J Med* 1993; **329**(18):1302–7
5 Rutgeerts P, Van Trappen G, Broeckaert L, et al. Palliative Nd:YAG laser therapy for cancer of the esophagus and gastroesophageal junction: impact on quality of remaining life. *Gastrointest Endosc* 1988;**34**:87.
6 Silvis SE, Farahmand M, Johnson JA, Ansel HJ, Ho SB. A randomized blinded comparison of omeprazole and ranitidine in the treatment of chronic esophageal stricture secondary to acid peptic esophagitis. *Gastrointest Endosc* 1996; **43**(3):216–21.

2 Vomiting

Definition

Acute nausea with or without vomiting is a common symptom and should be differentiated from gastro-oesophageal reflux . Nausea and vomiting result from a combination of physiological factors resulting from sensory input to the vomiting centre in the medulla or the chemoreceptor trigger zone (CTZ). The lower oesophageal sphincter relaxes and vomiting starts in the presence of a closed glottis.

Aetiology

The causes of acute nausea and vomiting are summarised in Table 2.1.

- *CNS causes* – these are associated with stimulation or disorders of the vestibular system, the commonest of which is motion sickness. Head injuries, intra-cranial inflammation and raised pressure are important factors.
- *Visceral* – visceral pain from a variety of intra-abdominal causes often associated with the acute abdomen including sepsis and mechanical obstruction. Gastric outlet obstruction leads to prolonged vomiting of the projectile type.
- *Drugs* – narcotics, cardiac glycoside and anti-cancer drugs. Paracetamol in overdose produces nausea but the commonest "recreational" cause is alcohol abuse.
- *Infections* – include epidemic viral infections, e.g. Norwalk agent, food poisoning.
- *Pregnancy*.

Table 2.1 Causes of acute vomiting.

CNS	Vestibular disorders CNS tumours Meningitis Reye's Syndrome Head injury Sub-arachnoid haemorrhage
Visceral stimuli	Peritonitis Small bowel obstruction Pseudo-obstruction Acute pancreatitis Acute cholecystitis Acute appendicitis Gastric outlet obstruction
Drugs	Chemotherapy drugs Antibiotics Digoxin Narcotics NSAIDs Aminophylline
Infectious	Sporadic viral infections Salmonella Hepatitis viruses
Miscellaneous	Psychogenic Diabetes Radiotherapy Pregnancy Carcinomatosis Uraemia

History

The main causes above should be considered when taking the history. A history of systemic symptoms of fever, myalgia, diarrhoea or possible infectious contacts in the family, school or workplace points to an infectious cause. In these situations, a stool sample may reveal Norwalk agent, *Salmonella*, *Staph. aureus* or *B.cereus*. If there are no obvious symptoms of infection, the female patient should be asked if she could be pregnant. A careful drug history may reveal the cause and the patient should be asked about recent relevant CNS symptoms of vertigo, headache, blurred vision or head injury. Recent symptoms of abdominal pain, anorexia or dyspepsia may suggest a visceral cause.

Examination

- Signs of dehydration – dry tongue, decreased skin turgor.

- Abdominal examination for signs of peritonism, gastric stasis, or acute intestinal obstruction.
- CNS signs of meningism, nystagmus, or papilloedema.
- Smell of alcohol or ketones on the breath.

Investigation

Investigations will be directed towards the suspected cause from the history.
If infection is suspected:

- stool culture.
- liver function tests.
- hepatitis serology.

If a visceral cause is suspected:

- In the presence of peritonism – plain abdominal radiographs may show an ileus, small bowel obstruction or free gas due to perforation.
- If biliary signs are present an abdominal ultrasound may show gallstones and a thickened gallbladder wall.
- Acute epigastric tenderness suggests acute pancreatitis and serum amylase is essential.
- Gastric outlet obstruction will be suggested by a succussion "splash" and should be confirmed by an endoscopy or barium meal *after* the residual gastric contents have been emptied using a naso-gastric tube.

If CNS causes suspected:

- Vestibular testing or a CT brain will be necessary. Lumbar puncture should be avoided until the presence of raised intra-cranial pressure has definitely been excluded.
- In all cases: urea and electrolytes, full blood count.

Management of acute nausea and vomiting

- *Fluid replacement.* If dehydration is present, and the patient cannot tolerate oral fluids, intravenous fluid replacement using normal saline should be started. Potassium supplements may be required in patients with gastric outlet obstruction or if the vomiting has been associated with prolonged diarrhoea
- *Specific anti-emetic drugs.* These agents are useful in the acute phase in the majority of cases of acute vomiting where the

underlying cause is not clear but urgent symptomatic relief is necessary. The main types of anti-emetic drugs are summarised in Table 2.2.

1   Prochlorperazine (Stemetil). Give 12·5 mg stat by deep im injection, followed by oral doses 10 mg 6-hourly prn if the vomiting is controlled. Beware of patients with Parkinson's disease, narrow angle glaucoma or a history of phenothiazine hypersensitivity.

2   Sublingual prochlorperazine maleate (Buccastem) 3 mg tablet can be placed high up between the upper lip and the gums to either side of the front teeth. Alternatively, a prochlorperazine suppository 25 mg can be placed per rectum stat followed by oral medication 6-hourly as above.

3   In patients where there is a contraindication to the above, Cyclizine hydrochloride, a histamine H1 receptor antagonist is effective. Give Cyclizine (Valoid) 50 mg by im injection. The drug will cause drowsiness and should be used in the elderly with caution.

4   If the first two drugs are not effective, the 5HT3 receptor antagonist Ondansetron (Zofran) should be given as a 4 mg dose either by im or slow iv injection. It can also be given as 16 mg suppositories. If vomiting is controlled after the initial dose, the oral form can be given in a dose up to 32 mg per day in the 4 or 8 mg tablet form.

Table 2.2 Classes of anti-emetic drug.

Anticholinergic	Scopolamine – for motion sickness/vest causes
Antihistamine	Promethazine, meclazine
Neuroleptics	Chlorpromazine, prochloperazine – useful in acute severe cases, drug induced cases and carcinomatosis
Prokinetic drugs	Metaclopramide Domperidone Cisapride – all useful in gastric dysmotility and of some symptomatic value in sporadic viral infections
5 HT3 antagonists	Ondansetron – effective in acute chemotherapy induced cases and resistant sporadic cases

3 Acute upper gastrointestinal haemorrhage

Natural history

Approximately 80% of upper gastrointestinal haemorrhage are self-limiting and require only supportive therapy. Patients with continued or recurrent bleeding have mortality rates of 30–40%.

Distinguishing upper from lower gastrointestinal haemorrhage

Upper gastrointestinal haemorrhage arises from above the ligament of Treitz while lower gastrointestinal haemorrhage arises from below this. Haematemesis is indicative of an upper gastrointestinal source. Melaena usually indicates upper gastrointestinal haemorrhage; this can result from as little as 50–100 ml of blood. In rare cases, melaena will occur from a lower gastrointestinal bleed, usually from the right colon. Bright red rectal bleeding usually indicates lower gastrointestinal haemorrhage. If this is arising from an upper source it requires at least 1000 ml of blood loss which is accompanied by haemodynamic instability. A transient rise in urea without a rise in creatinine suggests upper gastrointestinal haemorrhage.

Aetiology

Please see Table 3.1.

History

- Dyspepsia may indicate the diagnosis of an ulcer; alcohol excess suggests gastritis, Mallory–Weiss tear, or varices.

Table 3.1 Cause of upper gastrointestinal haemorrhage in 2225 patients.

Diagnoses	Percent of total diagnoses
Duodenal ulcer	24·3
Gastric erosions	23·4
Gastric ulcer	21·3
Varices	10·3
Mallory-Weiss tear	7·2
Oesophagitis	6·3
Erosive duodenitis	5·8
Neoplasm	2·9
Stomal ulcer	1·8
Oesophageal ulcer	1·7
Miscellaneous	6·8

Source: Silverstein FE, Gilbert DA, Tedesco FJ. The national ASGE survey on upper gastrointestinal bleeding. *Gastrointest Endsoc* 1981; **27**:73

- Ask about aspirin or NSAID drug ingestion.
- If there is a history of abdominal aortic aneurysm repair, an aortoenteric fistula must be considered.
- Collapse indicates a significant haemorrhage.
- Assess the presence or absence of comorbid disease.

Examination

- Assess the severity of the haemorrhage.
- An orthostatic decrease of 20 mm Hg in the systolic blood pressure or a postural increase in the pulse of 20 beats per minute is indicative of > 20% blood loss.
- With greater losses, resting pulse increases to > 100 beats per minute, systolic blood pressure falls to < 100 mm Hg followed by hypovolaemic shock.
- Stigmata of chronic liver disease suggests a diagnosis of varices.

Investigation
Bloods

- Check full blood count (may be misleading for several hours after the acute haemorrhage as redistribution of plasma from the extravascular to intravascular space occurs during the subsequent 24–72 h), coagulation profile, urea and electroytes, liver function tests.

- Send blood for group and hold if bleeding is not severe or cross match if bleeding is severe.

Management of acute upper gastrointestinal haemorrhage

Fluid replacement and resuscitation

- Large bore (14–18 gauge) intravenous cannulas should be placed for administration of fluids and blood products.
- A central venous pressure line may be helpful for estimating intravascular volume and judicious administration of fluids. A Swan–Ganz catheter may be used for patients with a history of unstable cardiovascular disease in whom accurate measurement of left ventricular filling pressure is necessary to prevent either over or insufficient fluid replacement.
- Consider intensive care support with haemodynamic monitoring if patient has adverse prognostic factors for upper gastrointestinal haemorrhage.
- Initial resuscitation is accomplished using normal saline if the patient's blood pressure is maintained or colloid if the patient is hypotensive until blood is available.
- If the haemoglobin or haematocrit is low, packed red blood cells are transfused. Whole blood or O negative blood if there is no time to cross-match is used if the patient is exsanguinating.
- Transfuse with blood until:
  - arterial pressure is greater than 80 mm Hg
  - heart rate less than 100 bpm
  - central venous pressure greater than 2 cm H20
  - haematocrit less than 25.
- Corrrect coagulopathy with fresh frozen plasma (3–5 units) if bleeding is severe.

Urinary catheter

- Patients should be catheterised to monitor their urine output.

Nasogastric tube and gastric lavage

- Gastric lavage may clear the stomach to facilitate endoscopic examination but there is a risk of aspiration, perforation or inadvertent placement into the respiratory tree and it delays endoscopy. Coagulation abnormalities should be corrected before this is performed. Most endoscopists do not perform lavage.

Triage

- Clinical prognostic factors can be used to decide whether the patient is admitted to an ordinary ward or intensive care unit (ICU) (See Table 3.2).
- The following factors are bad prognostic indicators and therefore put the patient in a high risk category where admission to ICU should be considered :
  - onset of haemorrhage in hospital
  - comorbid illnesses (cardiac, respiratory, renal, malignancy, neurological disease)
  - age >60
  - large transfusion requirement, especially if >4 units transfused.
- Patients considered low risk can be admitted to an ordinary ward.
- Endoscopic findings can be used to categorise the patient into high risk or low risk category (see Chapters 22 and 27).

Table 3.2 Rockall risk scoring system.

	0	1	2	3
Age	<60	60–79	<80	
Pulse	<100	>100		
SBP	<100	>100	<100	
Co-morbidity	None		IHD, CHF, any other	Renal or liver failure, malignancy
Diagnosis	Mallory-Weiss, no lesion, no stigmata	All others	UGI malignant lesions	
Stigmata	No or dark spot		Blood, clot, visible, spurting vessel	

Higher score, higher morbidity and mortality. If score < 2, risk of rebleeding is 4% and mortality < 0·1%. If score > 5, risk of rebleeding is > 24% and mortality > 11%.

18

Pharmacology

- Proton pump inhibitors may reduce rebleeding and surgery in those with peptic ulcer and stigmata of recent haemorrhage (conclusions from two of three randomised controlled trials).
- In these patients, proton pump inhibitors should be administered in standard doses, orally if the patient can manage this or by intravenous injection if the patient is nil by mouth.

Endoscopy

- The reasons for performing OGD include:
  - establishing a diagnosis
  - establishing prognosis (see Table 3.2 and Chapters 22 and 27)
  - therapy to either reduce risk of rebleeding or stop active bleeding, e.g. injection or coagulation therapy for peptic ulcer; sclerotherapy for oesophageal varices (see Chapters 22 and 27).
- OGD should be performed in all patients except:
  - young patients with minor haemorrhage associated with episodic alcohol use or gastroenteritis
  - terminally ill patients with minor bleeding.
- Prior to OGD, the following should be optimised and considered:
  - resuscitation of patient (see above). Their blood pressure should be stabilised if possible
  - initiation of medical therapy for unstable medical conditions, e.g. coagulopathy, arrhythmias, hypoxia. Coagulopathy is not a contraindication. Arrhythmias and hypoxia are contraindications
  - availability of skilled assistant, monitoring and therapeutic endoscopes and accessories (see Figure 3.1)
  - whether or not GI bleed has stopped or is ongoing.
- Timing of OGD:
  - urgent (as soon as possible after the above steps have been satisfied) in "high risk" patients (see above under Triage)
  - within 12–24 h in "low risk" patients.
- In those patients with massive bleeding, they should be intubated to protect their airway prior to OGD.
- Repeat endoscopy within 24 h should be considered in those with major stigmata of recent haemorrhage such as active bleeding or visible vessel.

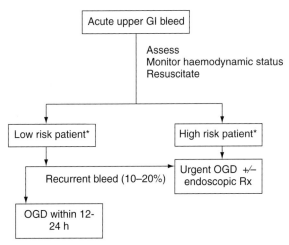

Figure 3.1 Approach to patient with acute upper GI bleed.* An estimate of risk can be made before endoscopy. Please see Table 3.2

Team approach

- In the high risk patients, both gastroenterologist and surgeon should be involved in the management.

Policy for rebleeding after endoscopic treatment

- Rebleeding is defined as recurrent bleeding occurring after initial successful endoscopic haemostasis.
- Signs of rebleeding are: haematemesis, tachycardia or fall in blood pressure or haemoglobin. Melaena per se is not a sign of rebleeding unless accompanied by tachycardia, fall in blood pressure or haemoglobin.
- In those who rebleed, repeat endoscopy and therapy should be attempted before surgical intervention.

Surgery

- The indications for urgent surgery are:
  - massive bleeding not stopped by endoscopic treatment
  - have recurrent bleeding despite endoscopic treatment.

Angiography

- This is used as a diagnostic and possibly therapeutic examination (accuracy 50–75%) only if endoscopy has failed to detect a source of bleeding. The bleeding must be arterial and at a rate of at least 0·5–0·6 ml/min to detect extravasation.

Feeding

- Patients should be on nil orally until endoscopy is performed. If the risk of rebleeding is low, patients should be allowed food immediately following endoscopy. If the risk of rebleeding is high, they should be kept on nil orally for a further 24 h.

Discharge home from hospital

- For risk of rebleeding, please see Table 3.2.
- Those with a low risk of rebleeding can be discharged as soon as they are stable following transfusion if necessary.
- Those with a high risk of rebleeding should remain in hospital for at least 72 h when the risk of rebleeding is highest.

Follow-up post discharge

- For those with peptic ulcers, please see Chapter 22.

Further reading

1 Consensus Development Panel. Consensus statement on therapeutic endoscopy and bleeding ulcers. *Gastrointest Endosc* 1990;**36**:S62–S65.
2 Daneshmend TK, Hawkey CJ, Langman MJ, Logan RF, Long RG, Walt RP. Omeprazole versus placebo for acute upper gastrointestinal bleeding: randomised double blind controlled trial. *BMJ* 1992;**304**(6820):143–7.
3 Griffin MR, Ray WA, Schaffner W. Nonsteroidal anti-inflammatory drug use and death from peptic ulcer in elderly patients. *Ann Intern Med* 1988;**109**:359–63.
4 Khuroo MS, Yattoo GN, Javid G, *et al.* A comparison of omeprazole and placebo for bleeding peptic ulcer. *N Engl J Med* 1997;**336**(15):1054–8.
5 Laine L. Multipolar electrocoagulation in the treatment of active upper gastrointestinal tract hemorrhage. A prospective controlled trial. *N Engl J Med* 1987;**316**(26):1613–17.
6 Rockall TA, Logan RF, Devlin HB, Northfield TC. Selection of patients for early discharge or outpatient care after acute upper gastrointestinal haemorrhage. National Audit of Acute Upper Gastrointestinal Haemorrhage. *Lancet* 1996;**347**(9009):1138–40.
7 Silverstein FE, Gilbert DA, Tedesco FJ, *et al.* The national ASGE survey of upper gastrointestinal bleeding. Part II. Clinical prognostic factors. *Gastrointest Endosc* 1981;**27**:80–93.

4 Acute abdominal pain

Introduction

Acute abdominal pain is a common gastro-intestinal emergency which may present to primary care physicians, gastroenterologists or surgeons. In the majority of cases in adults, the diagnosis can be established on clinical grounds without resort to extensive investigation.

Aetiology

The main causes of acute abdominal pain or "the acute abdomen" are shown in Table 4.1. The causes can be classified into:

- peritoneal (inflammatory haemorrhagic)
- obstructive
- miscellaneous.

Table 4.1 Causes of abdominal pain.

Infective/inflammatory	Acute cholecystitis
	Acute pancreatitis
	Acute appendicitis
	Pelvic inflammatory disease
Haemorrhagic	Ruptured aneurysm
	Ruptured ectopic pregnancy
	Mesenteric thrombosis
	Ruptured spleen
Obstructive	Intestinal obstruction
	Biliary obstruction
	Renal colic
Miscellaneous	Referred from chest, spine
	Diabetes
	Porphyria
	Psychogenic

Inflammation

This symptom complex is a consequence of an inflamed intra-abdominal viscus. The inflamed viscus causes irritation of the visceral peritoneum initially causing vague central abdominal pain which may be difficult for the patient to localise. Continued inflammation or localised perforation leads to involvement of the parietal peritoneum. Pain becomes localised and is then associated with tenderness, guarding and rebound tenderness on local palpation. Spread of infection generally throughout the abdominal cavity leads to generalised abdominal wall rigidity, often associated with a rigid or board-like abdomen. Generalised systemic signs of sepsis are at this stage with pyrexia, tachycardia and pallor.

Haemorrhagic

Although this is not the commonest cause of acute abdominal pain, it must be considered because of its serious and often rapid progression. It is due to bleeding into the peritoneal cavity or retroperitoneum either due to a leaking major vessel e.g. aortic aneurysm or a ruptured organ e.g. spleen or ectopic tubal pregnancy. Onset of the pain may be insidious and poorly localised at first. Soiling of the peritoneum with blood may simulate peritonitis. The bowel sounds may diminish and ileus may be present. The patient's circulatory system will show signs of shock and the abdomen will distend as bleeding progresses.

Obstructive

In this situation, a hollow viscus has a lumenal blockage which interferes with its normal motility pattern and its ability to deal with lumenal contents or secretions.

This results in often severe crampy pain as in cases of biliary colic where the cystic duct is obstructed by a gallstone or renal colic due to an obstructing uureteric calculus. When the bowel itself is obstructed the result is the classical clinical triad of:

- abdominal colic
- vomiting (due to failure of transit)
- increasing constipation.

Intestinal obstruction, if left untreated, will lead to perforation with signs of an acute abdomen. In the early stages of acute obstruction bowel sounds are often high pitched or "tinkling" in character but the sounds disappear when prolonged obstruction leads to perforation and peritonitis.

Non-specific acute abdominal pain

This presentation is common and may present with colicky abdominal pain or even progressive generalised pain. Pain may be a result from:

- parietal pleura in pneumonia
- sub-phrenic sepsis
- myocardial ischaemia
- due to diabetic ketoacidosis
- hypercalcaemia
- porphyria
- pschogenic factors.

In this scenario, the abdomen is usually generally tender with guarding. Bowel sounds are preserved and there are no signs of systemic sepsis or bleeding.

History

The four broad classifications of cause should be kept in mind and a careful history taken.

- Rapidity of onset – slow in obstruction and sepsis, fast in perforation and acute haemorrhage.
- Character of pain – constant or colicky .
- Associated abdominal symptoms – vomiting, diarrhoea.
- Systemic symptoms – fever, anorexia, fainting.
- Recent symptoms of dyspepsia, possible gallstone symptoms, amenorrhoea, dysuria or renal colic.
- Past history of peptic ulcer, gallstones, abdominal trauma or peripheral vascular disease (may point to aortic aneurysm).
- Drug history – recent NSAIDS or anticoagulants.
- History of diabetes, alcohol or drug abuse.

Examination

- The patient should be assessed for pyrexia, signs of shock, foetor and ketones on the breath.

- Light and deep palpation of the abdomen will indicate areas of local tenderness, rebound or guarding or whether generalised tenderness is present.
- Bruising in the flanks will indicate possible acute pancreatitis (see Chapter 23).
- A distended abdomen should suggest ascites which may be infected. Gas distension suggests obstruction.
- Bowel sounds will be high pitched in impending obstruction, absent in ileus or the presence of peritonitis.

Investigation

Several investigations are useful in cases of the acute abdomen.

- *Full blood picture and differential white cell count.* Haemoglobin will be reduced in the presence of acute intra-abdominal bleeding. White cell count will rise in the presence of sepsis with a neutrophilia in cases of bacterial infection.
- *Serum amylase* will be elevated in acute pancreatitis, perforated peptic ulcer and in some cases of ruptured abdominal aortic aneurysm.
- *Urea, electrolytes and blood glucose.* Sodium will be low in cases of pain associated with prolonged vomiting and decreased fluid intake.
- *Plain abdominal x ray (erect and supine)* will demonstrate bowel fluid levels in cases of obstruction, free intra-abdominal gas.
- *Chest x ray* may demonstrate a basal pneumonia or a pleural effusion.
- *Ultrasound of abdomen/contrast – enhanced CT* if ruptured aortic aneurysm, ectopic pregnancy or acute pancreatitis are suspected.

Treatment of specific causes of acute abdominal pain are dealt with in the specific sections relating to intra-abdominal emergencies.

5 Jaundice

Definition

Jaundice is the abnormal accumulation of bilirubin in body tissues which occurs when the serum bilirubin level exceeds 50 μmol/l (1.5 mg/dl). Excess bilirubin causes a yellow tinting to the skin, sclera, and mucous membranes.

Differential diagnosis

Conditions which cause jaundice can be classified under the broad categories of: (1) isolated disorder of bilirubin metabolism (*prehepatic jaundice*), (2) liver disease (*hepatic jaundice*) and (3) obstruction of the bile ducts (*obstructive jaundice*). See Table 5.1.

Table 5.1 Differential diagnosis of jaundice (common disorders are in *italics*).

Prehepatic jaundice: isolated disorders of bilirubin metabolism
Unconjugated hyperbilirubinaemia
1 Increased bilirubin production, e.g. *haemolysis, ineffective erythropoeisis*, blood transfusion, resorption of haematomas
2 Decreased hepatocellular uptake, e.g. rifampicin
3 Decrease conjugation, e.g. *Gilbert's syndrome*, Crigler-Najjar syndrome, physiologic jaundice of the newborn

Conjugated or mixed hyperbilirubinaemia
1 Dubin-Johnson syndrome
2 Rotor's syndrome

Hepatic jaundice: liver disease
Acute or chronic hepatocellular dysfunction
1 Acute or subacute
   ● *Viral hepatitis*
   ● Toxins (*alcohol*, amanita),

- Drugs (*paracetamol*, isoniazid, methyldopa)
- Ischaemia (hypotension, vascular occlusion)
- Metabolic disorders (Wilson's disease, Reye's syndrome),
- Pregnancy related (acute fatty liver of pregnancy, pre-eclampsia)

2 Chronic
  - *Viral hepatitis*
  - Toxins (*ethanol*, vinyl chloride, vitamin A)
  - *Autoimmune hepatitis*
  - Metabolic (*Haemachromatosis*, Wilson's disease, α1-antitrypsin deficiency)

Obstructive jaundice: obstruction of the bile ducts

Extrahepatic
1 *Choledocholithiasis*
2 Diseases of the bile ducts
  - Neoplasms (*cholangiocarcinoma*)
  - Inflammation/infection (primary sclerosing cholangitis, AIDS cholangiopathy, hepatic arterial chemotherapy, post-surgical strictures)
3 Extrinsic compression of the biliary tree
  - Neoplasms (*pancreatic carcinoma*, metastatic lymphadenopathy, hepatoma)
  - Chronic pancreatitis
  - Vascular enlargement (aneurysm, portal cavernova)

Intrahepatic: hepatic disorders with prominent cholestasis
1 Diffuse infiltrative disorders
  - Granulomatous diseases (mycobacterial infections, *sarcoidosis*, *lymphoma*, drug toxicity, Wegener's granulomatosis)
  - Amyloidosis
  - Malignancy
2 Inflammation of intrahepatic bile ductules and/or portal tracts
  - *Primary biliary cirrhosis*
  - Graft-versus-host disease
  - Drug toxicity (*chlorpromazine, erythromycin*)
3 Miscellaneous
  - Benign recurrent intrahepatic cholestasis
  - Drug toxicity
  - Oestrogens, anabolic steroids
  - Total parenteral nutrition
  - Bacterial infections
  - Uncommon manifestations of viral or alcoholic hepatitis
  - Intrahepatic cholestasis of pregnancy
  - Postoperative cholestasis

History and examination

An algorithm for assessing the patient with jaundice is shown in Figure 5.1. The history and examination provide important clues regarding the cause of the jaundice. See Table 5.2.

A simplified aide memoire to help remember to ask specific questions to ascertain the cause of jaundice is as follows:

A alcohol
B blood transfusion

27

C contact with jaundice
D drugs
E environment
F foreign travel, family history
G gallstones
H hepatitis.

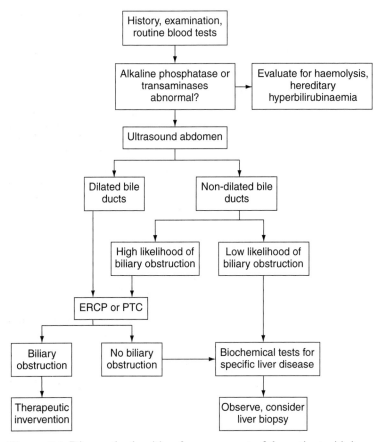

Figure 5.1 Diagnostic algorithm for assessment of the patient with jaundice (From Lidofsky S, Scharschmidt BF. Jaundice. In: Feldman M, Scharschmidt BF, Sleisenger MH eds. *Gastrointestinal and liver disease*, 6th edn. Philadelphia: WB Saunders. 1998:200–32, with permission.)

Table 5.2 Differentiating obstructive jaundice from hepatic jaundice.

Suggests obstructive jaundice	Suggests hepatic jaundice
History	
Abdominal pain	Anorexia, malaise, myalgias, viral-type
Fever, rigors	illness
Prior biliary surgery	Known infectious exposure
Older age	Receipt of blood products, use of
Dark urine and pale stools	intravenous drugs
	Exposure to known hepatotoxin
	Family history of jaundice
Physical examination	
High fever	Ascites
Abdominal tenderness	Stigmata of liver disease (e.g.
Palpable abdominal mass	gynaecomastia, spider naevi, Kayser-
Abdominal scar	Fleischer rings
Urinalysis – large amount of bilirubin	Asterixis, encephalopathy
with little or no urobilinogen	Urinalysis – mixture of bilirubin and
	urobilinogen
Laboratory Tests	
Predominant elevation of serum bilirubin	Predominant elevation of serum
and alkaline phosphatase	transaminases
Prothrombin time that is normal or	Prothrombin time that does not
normalises with vitamin K administration	correct with vitamin K administration
Elevated serum amylase	Blood tests indicative of specifice liver
	disease, e.g. autoantibodies, positive
	viral serology

Source: Lidofsky S, Scharschmidt BF. Jaundice. In: Feldman M, Scharschmidt BF, Sleisenger MH, eds. *Sleisenger and Fordtran's gastrointestinal and liver disease*, 6th edn. Philadelphia: WB Saunders, 1998:220–32.

Investigations
Blood tests
The following bloods should be performed:

- liver function tests – bilirubin, alkaline phosphatase, transaminases (AST and ALT), gamma – GT, albumin
- prothrombin time
- hepatitis A, B, C serology
- auto-antibody screen – mitochondrial, smooth muscle, nuclear; (liver, kidney, microsomal)
- immunoglobulins
- iron studies.

The following bloods should be considered if history or physical exam suggests this:

- alpha1-antitrypsin – if deficiency is considered
- copper and caeruloplasmin – if Wilson's disease is considered

Ultrasound scan

This determines the calibre of the extrahepatic biliary tree and reveals mass lesions. The sensitivity of abdominal ultrasound for the detection of biliary obstruction in jaundiced patients ranges from 55–91% and the specificity from 82–95%. It can demonstrate cholelithiasis. Common duct stones may not be seen; the negative predictive value of a dilated duct seen on scan with no stones seen is about 50% for actual common duct stones. The positive predictive value of a dilated duct with ductal stones seen on scan is about 90%. Ultrasound can detect space-occupying lesions greater than 1 cm in diameter.

Computed tomography

CT is not as accurate as ultrasound in detecting cholelithiasis. It can detect space-occupying lesions as small as 5 mm. It provides technically superior images to ultrasound in obese patients and those in whom the biliary tree is obscured by bowel gas. Its accuracy for detecting biliary obstruction is similar to ultrasound. CT with intravenous contrast material can evaluate the aetiology of biliary obstruction such as stone or stricture.

Endoscopic retrograde cholangiopancreatography (ERCP) (see Chapter 12)

It is highly accurate in the diagnosis of biliary obstruction with a sensitivity of 89–98% and specificity of 89–100%. Biopsy specimens, brushings for cytology can be obtained. If a focal cause for biliary obstruction such as a stone or stricture is detected, then therapeutic maneouvres to relieve the obstruction such as sphincterotomy, stone extraction, dilatation, stent placement can be performed during the same session. However it is invasive with a risk of complications in about 10% (pancreatitis, haemorrhage, perforation, cholangitis).

Percutaneous transhepatic cholangiography (PTC)

PTC requires the passage of a needle through the skin into the hepatic parenchyma and peripheral bile duct. The sensitivity and specificity are comparable to ERCP. PTC may be technically more difficult in the absence of intrahepatic duct dilatation. Therapeutic procedures such as stent placement can be performed. However bile duct stones cannot be easily extracted. There is a risk of complications (bleeding, perforation, cholangitis, bile leak).

Magnetic resonance cholangiography (MRC)

In a few series, the accuracy of MR cholangiography approached that of ERCP. Although promising, its exact role in the diagnostic evaluation of jaundice is as yet undefined.

Liver Biopsy

Liver biopsy provides information regarding hepatic lobular architecture and is most helpful in patients with undiagnosed persistent jaundice. It permits the diagnosis of viral hepatitis, alcoholic hepatitis, Wilson's disease, haemochromatosis, alpha1-antitrypsin deficiency, fatty liver of pregnancy, primary biliary cirrhosis, granulomatous hepatitis, neoplasms. It may provide clues to unsuspected biliary tract obstruction. There is a small complication rate (bleeding and perforation) of about 1.7% (see Chapter 14).

Management of jaundice

Biliary obstruction

Therapy is directed at the mechanical relief of obstruction. The options include ERCP (sphincterotomy, stone extraction, stent insertion), PTC (stent insertion) or surgery. The therapeutic strategy depends on the likely aetiology and local expertise.

Hepatic jaundice

The therapy is directed towards the underlying aetiology, e.g. stopping alcohol, discontinuation of a drug, antiviral agents, phlebotomy for haemochromatosis, copper chelation for Wilson's.

Pruritus

The pruritogen is thought to be a bile acid, bile acid derivative or some other substance that undergoes enterohepatic circulation. Drugs which may be helpful include:

- cholestyramine
- antihistamines
- ursodeoxycholic acid (especially in primary biliary cirrhosis)
- phenobarbital
- rifampicin.

Further reading

1 Carr-Locke DL, Cotton PB. Biliary tract and pancreas. *Br Med Bull* 1986;**42**(3):257–64.
2 Gilmore IT, Burroughs A, Murray-Lyon IM, Williams R, Jenkins D, Hopkins A. Indications, methods, and outcomes of percutaneous liver biopsy in England and Wales: an audit by the British Society of Gastroenterology and the Royal College of Physicians of London. *Gut* 1995;**36**(3):437–41
3 Lidofsky S, Scharschmidt BF. Jaundice. In: Feldman M, Scharschmidt BF, Sleisenger MD, eds. *Gastrointestinal and liver disease*, 2nd edn. Philadelphia: WB Saunders, 1998.
4 Richter JM, Silverstein MD, Schapiro R. Suspected obstructive jaundice: a decision analysis of diagnostic strategies. *Ann Intern Med* 1983;**99**:46.
5 Teplick SK, Flick P, Brandon JC. Transhepatic cholangiography in patients with suspected biliary disease and nondilated intrahepatic bile ducts. *Gastrointest Radiol* 1991;**16**:193.

6 Acute lower gastrointestinal haemorrhage

with contributions from John Moorehead, Paul Neilly

Introduction

Lower gastrointestinal haemorrhage is defined as bleeding arising from beyond the second part of duodenum and accounts for approximately 5% of emergency hospital admissions. Most patients are elderly with associated co-morbidity making investigation and definitive management difficult but bleeding usually stops spontaneously (80% of cases). A major bleed may be defined as a loss of >15% blood volume or requirement of >2 units of blood over the first 24 h.

Aetiology

The causes of lower gastrointestinal haemorrhage are summarised in Table 6.1 with colorectal and anal lesions account for 85% of acute bleeds.

History

Differentiation between upper and lower gastrointestinal bleeding can be difficult. This is discussed in Chapter 3.

Examination

In the otherwise fit patient tachycardia, tachypnoea and decrease in pulse pressure suggest a 15–30% acute blood loss (800–1500 ml). A measurable fall in systolic blood pressure indicates >30% reduction in circulating blood volume (>1500 ml). In these patients resuscitation is the priority and should be instituted before further investigation and definitive management.

33

Table 6.1 Aetiology of lower gastrointestinal haemorrhage.

Condition	Cause of haemorrhage
Congenital abnormalities	Meckel's diverticulum
Vascular changes	Angiodysplasia Arteriovenous malformation Telangectasia Haemorrhoids Rectal/colonic varices Vasculitis Aortoenteric fistula
Ischaemia	Ischaemic colitis Mesenteric ischaemia Necrotizing enterocolitis Marathon runner's colon
Dysentry	Bacterial (salmonellosis, shigellosis, *E. coli enterocolitis, Campylobacter colitis, Yersinia enterocolitis*) Parasitic (amoebiasis, giardiasis, schistosomiasis)
Neoplasia	Haemangioma Leiomyoma/leiomyosarcoma Polyps (adenoma, hyperplastic, hamartoma) Colorectal cancer
Inflammation	Ulcerative colitis/Crohn's disease Radiation enterocolitis/proctitis Henoch–Schönlein purpura
Trauma	Surgery Endoscopic polypectomy
Structural abnormality	Diverticulosis *Pneumatosis coli* Collagen disorders (Ehlers–Danlos syndrome, pseudoxanthoma elasticum) Endometriosis Dieulafoy's lesion
Pharmacological	Anticoagulants Non-steroidal anti-inflammatory drugs Cytotoxic chemotherapy

Abdominal examination indicates focal areas of tenderness (diverticulitis, Crohn's disease), palpable masses (colonic tumours, Crohn's disease) and organomegaly (secondary intestinal cancer, lymphoma). Digital anal examination may identify anal fissures, haemorrhoids or rectal tumours.

Investigations

Blood tests

All patients require a full blood picture and coagulation screen. Those with major haemorrhage (estimated loss >750 ml) and/or hypovolaemia/anaemia (haemoglobin <10 g/dl) should have blood crossmatched with at least 2 units held in reserve.

Urea and electrolytes should be performed.

Proctoscopy or sigmoidoscopy

This is essential in all these patients to exclude easily visualised anorectal causes of bleeding such as haemorrhoids, proctitis, tumours/polyps and solitary rectal ulcer.

Identification of bleeding source

- When bleeding from the upper gastrointestinal tract has been excluded and proctoscopy or sigmoidoscopy is unhelpful; *colonoscopy, isotope scanning and mesenteric angiography* should be considered.
- The advantages and disadvantages of each of these methods are summarised in Table 6.2.
- The best initial investigation is colonoscopy unless there is active bleeding in which case angiography is best.
- If colonoscopy fails to detect the cause for bleeding, then angiography should be considered if bleeding is brisk or isotope scan if bleeding is slow.
- A combination of tests (e.g. isotope scanning followed by angiography or colonoscopy) can provide more precise information allowing planning of further non-operative/operative measures.
- *Enteroscopy* is indicated for those with obscure bleeding beyond the reach of the standard endoscope. Diagnostic accuracy is >50% and the yield is maximised using video enteroscopes.

Management of acute lower gastrointestinal haemorrhage (see Figure 6.1)

Fluid resuscitation

- Large bore intravenous cannulas (14 G) and urinary catheters should be inserted and fluid administration started immediately.
- The volume of fluid and blood transfusion is titrated according to the clinical impression of blood loss (based on history,

Table 6.2 Investigations for gastrointestinal haemorrhage – advantages and disadvantages.

Procedure	Advantages	Disadvantages
Angiography	Good localisation of bleed Indicates rate of bleed Demonstrates pathology (e.g. AV malformation/ angiodysplasia) May be used intraoperatively (methylene blue test) Therapeutic (vasopressin, embolisation)	Requires fast bleeding (>1ml/min) Operator dependant Procedure related morbidity (9%)
Isotope scan	Detects slow bleeds (0.05-0.1ml/min) Safe Minimally invasive Specifically identifies Meckel's diverticulum (^{99m}Tc labelled pertechnetate)	Poor localisation of bleed Doesn't identify cause of bleed Liver, spleen, large vessels may overshadow site of bleeding Not readily available in many hospitals May require prolonged scanning
Colonoscopy	Can give good localisation May demonstrate pathology Therapeutic potential (electro-/laser coagulation, polypectomy) May be used intraoperatively	Technically difficult with active bleeding (~50% success) Operator dependant Risk of perforation

haemodynamic status, urinary output and visual loss), haemoglobin concentration and packed cell volume.

- With massive haemorrhage (>1500 ml) and in the elderly central venous pressure measurement will often be necessary.
- Successful resuscitation is indicated by warm peripheries, normal pulse rate and blood pressure, central venous pressure >10 mm Hg, urinary output >0·5 ml/kg/h and haemoglobin concentration >10 g/dl. When stable these patients can be formally investigated as discussed above.

Angiography

- This is useful in brisk haemorrhage where colonoscopy may not be able to detect a bleeding lesion.
- Angiodysplasias can be treated by embolisation or administration of intra-arterial vasopressin

Colonoscopy

- Bowel preparation with oral polyethylene glycol or Fleet

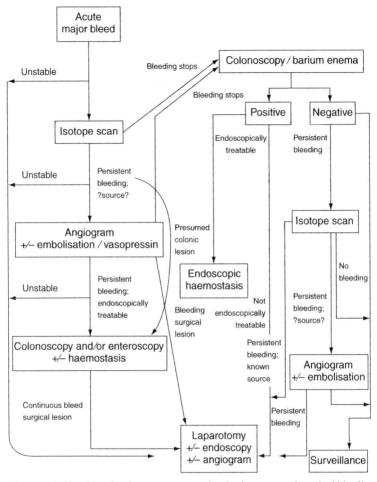

Figure 6.1 Algorithm for the management of major lower gastrointestinal bleeding.

Phosphosoda should be performed even with continuing haemorrhage.

- Colonoscopy can treat lesions causing lower gastrointestinal haemorrhage such as diverticular bleeding or angiodysplasia by coagulating or injecting the bleeding vessel.

Surgery

- Patients with massive haemorrhage should be considered for an emergency laparotomy.

- If the bleeding source cannot be identified intraoperatively a colectomy with ileorectal anastomosis is advised.

Further reading

1 Beck DE. Hemorrhoidal disease. In: Beck DE, Wexner SD, eds. *Fundamentals of anorectal surgery*. London: WB Saunders, 1998: 237–53.
2 Carter DC. Non-neoplastic structural disease of the colon. In: Shearman DJC, Finlayson NDC, Camilleri M, Carter DC, eds. *Diseases of the gastrointestinal tract and liver*. London: Churchill Livingstone, 1997: 1379–98.
3 Demarkles MP, Murphy JR. Acute lower gastrointestinal bleeding. *Med Clin N Am* 1993;**73**: 1085–100.
4 Forbes A, ed. *Clinicians' guide to inflammatory bowel disease*. London: Chapman & Hall, 1997.
5 Foutch PG. Angiodysplasia of the gastrointestinal tract. Am J Gastroenterol 1993;**88**(6): 807–18.
6 Keighley MRB. Bleeding from the colon and rectum. In: Keighley MRB, Williams NS, eds. *Surgery of the anus, rectum and colon*. London: WB Saunders, 1993: 1926–70.
7 Lewis BS. Small intestinal bleeding. *Gastroenterol Clin N Am* 1994;**23**:67–91.
8 Phillips RKS, ed. *A companion to specialist surgical practice: colorectal surgery*. London: WB Saunders, 1998.
9 Vernava AM III, Moore BA, Longo WE, Johnson FE. Lower gastrointestinal bleeding. *Dis Colon Rectum* 1997;**40**(7): 846–58.

7 Diarrhoea

Definition

Diarrhoea is defined as a decrease in consistency or increased liquidity of the stool. Some definitions also include increased frequency of defaecation and increased daily stool weight in the definition but these criteria have been limited by normal variation within a patient population. Acute diarrhoea is usually defined as persistence of symptoms for at least 2–3 weeks.

Differential diagnosis

Acute diarrhoea can be classified according to its underlying physiological mechanisms (Table 7.1).

Osmotic diarrhoea results from the presence of poorly absorbed solutes within the gut lumen leading to a net loss of water and usually large volumes of watery faeces are passed daily.

Secretory diarrhoea is caused by disturbed absorption of water and electrolytes in the presence of gut mucosal disease or inflammatory mediators. It may also occur in situations where the gut mucosa becomes a net loser of ions and water.

Dysmotility diarrhoea is caused by increase transit time of lumenal contents, bacterial overgrowth due to stasis and is probably compounded by ano-rectal dysfunction.

Inflammatory or exudative diarrhoea as the term suggests is the result of an acute inflammatory insult to the mucosa which may be idiopathic such as ulcerative colitis or associated with an infecting micro-organism. This type is usually associated with the passage of blood, mucous and white bood cells.

The differential of acute diarrhoea is summarised in Table 7.2.

Table 7.1 Physiological mechanisms in acute diarrhoea.

Mechanism	Disorder
Osmotic	Disaccharide deficiencies Magnesium induced Short bowel Extensive mucosal disease, e.g. coeliac, Crohn's Bile salt malabsorption Pancreatic insufficiency
Secretory	Toxins, e.g. cholera, clostridium Excess gut hormones Stimulant laxatives Bacterial overgrowth Inflammatory bowel disease Diabetic neuropathy Villous adenoma of the rectum Carcinoma of the rectum
Dysmotility	Functional bowel disease Endocrine disorders Autonomic neuropathies
Inflammatory	Infections Inflammatory bowel disease Ischaemic bowel disease

Table 7.2 Differential diagnosis of acute diarrhoea.

Cause	Remarks
Infections	Viral – adenovirus, astrovirus, calicivirus, rotavirus Bacterial-*Salmonella* spp., *Shigella* spp., *E. coli* spp. Parasites – Entamoeba histolytica, Giardia lamblia Food related – *Bacillus cereus*, *Staphylococcal* spp. Toxins - *Clostridia* spp.
Inflammatory bowel disease	Ulcerative colitis Crohn's disease Colitis indeterminate Collagenous colitis
Ischaemic colitis	
Drugs	Antibiotics ACE inhibitors Digoxin Chemotherapeutic agents Lipid lowering drugs Prostaglandin analogues PPI's Magnesium containing antacids
Faecal impaction	

History

- In the clinical history it is important to establish the following facts:
  - that diarrhoea is definitely present (as defined above)
  - rapidity of onset, frequency and whether sleep disturbed
  - presence of blood
  - presence of abdominal pain
  - recent drug, travel, dietary and sexual history
  - presence of vomiting/systemic symptoms and fever
  - prior history of irritable bowel/inflammatory bowel disease.
- The passage of stool volumes >1000 ml daily suggests a secretory process, while the pattern of <500 ml daily with moderate frequency of 5–8 stools is more likely to represent a motility abnormality.
- The presence of blood should always point to the presence of an acute inflammatory process sometimes due to an infecting agent.
- Bulky, pale, large volume stools which are difficult to flush suggest that significant fat malabsorption is the underlying problem and may point to a diagnosis of small bowel mucosal disease, pancreatic insufficiency or bacterial overgrowth.

Examination

Careful clinical examination may yield important clues to the cause of the diarrhoea in some patients. In general, it is important to assess for:

1. Signs of dehydration and circulatory collapse due to water and electrolyte depletion-tachycardia, hypotension, decreased skin turgor and dry mucus membranes.
2. Abdominal signs of an acute colitic or ischaemic process – abdominal mass, tenderness, guarding or rebound.
3. Rectal signs of bleeding on pr examination

- Certain general signs may point to a cause.
  - Evidence of thyrotoxicosis.
  - Collagen disease.
  - The skin signs associated with inflammatory bowel disease – pyoderma gangrenosus, erythema nodosum.
  - Dermatitis herpetiformis due to coeliac disease.
  - Flushing, wheeze and pulmonary stenosis due to carcinoid syndrome.

- Signs of peripheral vascular disease.
- Signs of diabetic complications.

Investigation

- Acute diarrhoea is very common in the community, often occurring in isolated outbreaks associated with enteric viral infections. Most cases are diagnosed in the Primary Care setting on clinical grounds without resort to sophisticated investigation. However a proportion of cases where the symptoms are prolonged, associated with systemic illness or rectal bleeding are referred for further hospital assessment as outpatients or acute admissions.
- The following investigations are likely to lead to a rapid diagnosis in the majority of cases:
  - Fresh stool sample for culture and sensitivity, occult blood, ova, cysts and parasites, c difficile toxin and giardia antigen.
  - Full blood count and DWCC.
  - Urea and electrolytes.
  - ESR, C reactive protein, alpha 1 antiglobulin.
  - Blood culture if pyrexia/rigors.
  - Rigid sigmoidoscopy, biopsy if indicated.
  - Plain x ray abdomen.
  - Flexible sigmoidoscopy proceeding to colonoscopy may be indicated in some cases.
  - Duodenal aspirates.

Management of acute diarrhoea

In all cases the management has three important components:

1 Correction of systemic electrolyte disturbance, anaemia and nutritional abnormalities which have arisen as a direct result of the acute illness. This is of particular importance in the frail elderly and children.
2 Oral rehydration solutions (see Table 7.3), which were initially developed for fluid replacement in dehydrated patients with cholera, are useful in the treatment of severe acute diarrhoea in all age groups, provided an oral intake is tolerated
3 If an infecting pathogen is detected in stools or less commonly, in blood cultures consideration should be given to specific antimicrobial therapy. The following points apply.

- In the absence of systemic features, antibiotics should be

Table 7.3 Oral rehydration solutions.

WHO/UNICEF Solution

 Contains Na 90 mmol/l, K 20 mmol/l , Cl 80 mmol/l, Bicarbonate 30 mmol/l and glucose 111 mmol/l

 It can be mixed readily in the hospital pharmacy

Dioralyte

 This commercial preparation contains Na 35 mmol/l, K 20 mmol/l, Cl 37 mmol/l, bicarbonate 18 mmol/l and glucose 200 mmol/l.

 These solutions may be given by naso-gastric tube feed if necessary until the diarrhoea has settled

---

avoided as most cases of enteric infection are self-limiting and do not require specific anti-microbial therapy.

- Anti-diarrhoeal agents may delay enteric clearance of pathogens and should be avoided if possible unless symptoms are very severe (see Chapter 37).

4 Infective causes of acute diarrhoea may closely mimic acute inflammatory bowel disease and should be ruled out by stool culture *before* steroid therapy is started.

Specific treatment

Specific treatment of diarrhoea is discussed in Chapters 35 and 37.

Part II
Complications of
gastrointestinal procedures

8 Introduction to section

There have been many major advances in gastrointestinal procedures over the years. These procedures provide valuable diagnostic information and in many cases have therapeutic potential
such as endoscopic removal of bile duct stones and treatment of
variceal bleeding. All procedures are associated with risk. However
the incidence of complications is low and in many instances quite
uncommon and is outweighed by the benefits of doing the procedure. The discussion of the benefits of the procedures is beyond the
scope of this book and it is hoped that the risk of complications is
not over-emphasised but put into its right context of benefits versus risk consideration.

9 Upper gastrointestinal endoscopy

Introduction

Large scale studies in the UK and the US have emphasised that oesophago-gastro-duodenoscopy (OGD) is associated with a very low complication rate. A large American survey in 1974 reported an overall complication rate of 0·13%, while a UK study in 1978 reported a complication rate of 0·1%.

Complications

- Sedation.
- Haemorrhage.
- Perforation of the pharynx, oesophagus, stomach or douodenum.

Complications of sedation

Clinical features

Although there is an ongoing trend towards the avoidance of sedation for OGD in some countries, intravenous sedation with benzodiazepines and pethidine is still widely used especially in therapeutic procedures such as variceal sclerotherapy or stricture dilatation.

Benzodiazepines can cause repiratory depression leading to apnoea. Hypotension is a potential adverse effect of midazolam which is four times more potent than diazepam on an iv dosage basis. Pethidine is a predominant narcotic analgesic with mild sedative properties. It is mainly used for potentialy painful procedures. The duration of action is 2–3 h. Overdosage can lead to cardio-pulmonary depression, nausea, vomiting and urinary retention. Adverse drug reactions have been reported in conjunction with MAOI drugs which should be stopped 14 days before administration.

Patients at risk from accidental over-sedation are the frail elderly, those with pre-existing cardio-pulmonary or hepatic disease and patients already on oral sedatives, phenothiazines and opiates.

Management

- *Reversal agents.* Flumezanil (*Anexate*) is a competitive benzodiazepam antagonist which effectively reverses their sedative action in doses of 200–400 mcg over 5 min when given iv. Episodes of rebound sedation do occur and repeated administration may be required up to a maximum dose of 1 mg.

  Naloxone (*Narcan*) reverses the respiratory depressant effects of pethidine in a dosage of 0·4–0·8 mg given iv. The dosages can be repeated slowly up to a maximum of 10 mg.

- *Safe sedation during endoscopy.* The specialist gastroenterology societies along with the Royal Colleges of Surgery and Anaesthetics have provided clear safety guidelines devised to minimise complications of over sedation. These include:
  - Endoscopy must only be performed with close patient monitoring of vital signs, including pulse oximetry.
  - If iv sedation is being used an indwelling plastic cannula should be placed.
  - Full rescuscitation equipment should be available in the endoscopy room with the appropriate reversal drugs.
  - Sedative drug doses should be slowly titrated according to patient consciousness levels and according to perceived needs, always taking risk factors into account levels and according to perceived needs, always taking risk factors into account.

Haemorrhage

Clinical features

This is a rare complication of diagnostic OGD but it may be encountered if the endoscope accidentally causes mucosal trauma or if a biopsy site bleeds either immediately in the aftermath of the procedure. Patients on anticoagulants probably have an increased risk due to trauma and biopsies should not be taken in these cases without adequate prior correction of the prothrombin time.

Haemorrhage at the time of OGD will be easily recognised but the site may not be clear especially if the bleeding is from the oropharynx or brisk gastro – duodenal bleeding obscures mucosal detail.

Management:

- If the bleeding site is in the stomach or duodenum and easily identified, it should be injected with 1:10000 adrenaline or coagulated with a BICAP probe or an Argon Plasma Coagulator if available. Minor oozing may settle after spraying the same adrenaline solution topically on to the mucosa.
- Brisk bleeding which obscures the view is rare in the diagnostic scenario. In these situations, the therapeutic options include; injecting or coagulating the site of bleeding endoscopically to stop the bleed, considering surgery or adopting a conservative approach in the expectation that the bleeding may stop spontaneously.
- An intravenous line should be erected
- Blood should be sent for urgent Group and cross-match and coagulation screen.
- Intravenous proton pump inhibitor (omeprazole or pantoprazole) should be given.
- The patients condition should be closely monitored.
- Only in rare situations will surgical intervention be required but a repeat check endoscopy should be arranged within 24 h or earlier if the patient is unstable.

Perforation

Management of perforation of the oesophagus is discussed in Chapter 16.

Management of perforation of the stomach and duodenum is discussed in Chapter 17.

Infection

Infection introduced at upper GI endoscopy is very rare. A transient bacteraemia is possible and could be a risk factor for bacterial endocarditis in patients with valvular heart disease or a prosthetic valve. Current recommendations from the American Society for Gastrointestinal Endoscopy do not recommend routine antibiotic prophylaxis for diagnostic upper GI endoscopy but prophlaxis should be given where the patient is undergoing:

- variceal injection
- oesophageal stricture dilatation.

Thirty minutes prior to endoscopy, the patient should be given amoxycillin 1 g and gentamicin 60 mg iv stat, then oral amonycillin 500 mg 6 h later. For patients who are allergic to penicillin, vancomycin IG over 100 minutes is given iv instead of amonycillin.

10 PEG

Introduction

Since the first descriptions of this technique by Gauderer and colleagues over 20 years ago, percutaneous endoscopic gastrostomy (PEG) is now a widely accepted alternative to naso-gastric tube feeding in patients with long term swallowing disorders.

The major complication rate is 1·0–4·0% for this procedure. It is important to assess those patients for whom PEG placement is *relatively* contraindicated:

- ascites
- morbid obesity
- gastric varices
- gastric mass
- proximal small bowel fistula.

Absolute contraindications include:

- unco-operative patients
- active sepsis
- oesophageal or gastric outlet obstruction
- incorrectable coagulopathy
- patient unfit for endoscopy.

Although the complication rate is quite low overall and the procedure-related mortality is less than 1%, major complications are associated with a 25% mortality when they do occur.

Minor complications related to the PEG tube such as leakage or stomal enlargement are not encountered as emergencies and the following section will deal with major complications.

Complications

Bronchial aspiration

Clinical features

Due to their relative age, frail state and co-morbid diseases PEG patients have an incidence of acute aspiration of 0·7% in the first 24 h after placement.

Symptoms and signs include fever, cough, dyspnoea and *x* ray changes of patchy basal consolidation.

Management

Measures which may help to decrease the incidence of aspiration include:

- Raise bedhead for 1–2 h after feeds.
- Drain stomach for 24 h before commencing first feeds to allow for ileus.
- Start feeding with small amounts and increase as tolerated.
- Broad spectrum antibiotics and chest physiotherapy if aspiration occurs.

Bleeding

Clinical features:

This complication has been reported in 2·5% of patients and is usually caused by pressure-induced mucosal ulceration beneath the intra-gastric retaining sponge or "bumper" (Figure 10.1).

The patient will present with haematemesis and/or melaena a few days after the procedure. There may be an unexplained drop in haemoglobin in the absence of overt signs.

Management

- At placement the bumper should not be pulled too tightly against the anterior gastric wall.
- The patient should be endoscoped if the bleeding persists or is major.
- At endoscopy, the PEG tube should be pushed in so that the area under the bumper can be carefully examined and any bleeding point injected with 1:10 000 adrenaline.
- The tube should be fixed in its new position on the abdominal wall to prevent further mucosal trauma.
- Start proton pump inhibitor therapy to accelerate healing.

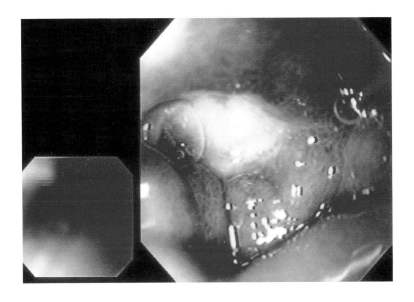

Plate 1 Acute duodenal ulcer with a clean base. Risk of rebleeding is 0–3%.

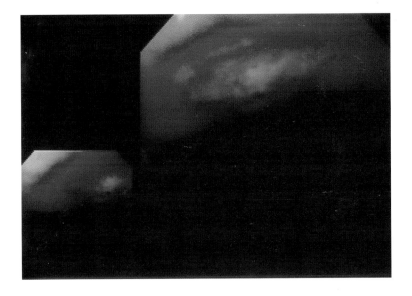

Plate 2 Acute gastric ulcer with a flat spot. Risk of rebleeding is 5–10%.

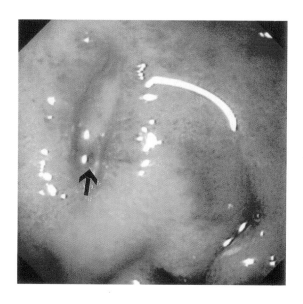

Plate 3 Acute duodenal ulcer with a visible vessel (arrow). Risk of rebleeding is 50%.

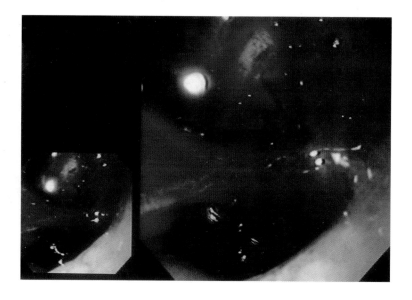

Plate 4 Acute duodenal ulcer with an adherent clot. Risk of rebleeding is 30%.

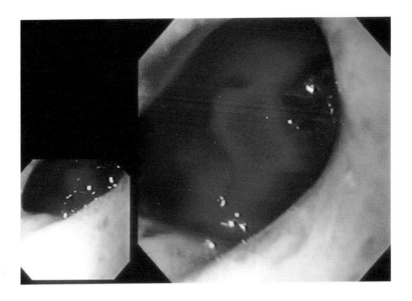

Plate 5 Same acute duodenal ulcer in Plate 4 with active arterial bleeding. Risk of rebleeding is 90–100%.

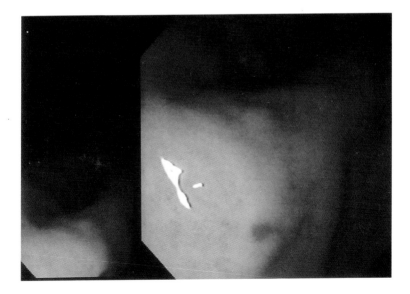

Plate 6 Telangiectatic lesion in body of stomach. There are fine spidery "tentacles" around the periphery that distinguish it from scope trauma artefact.

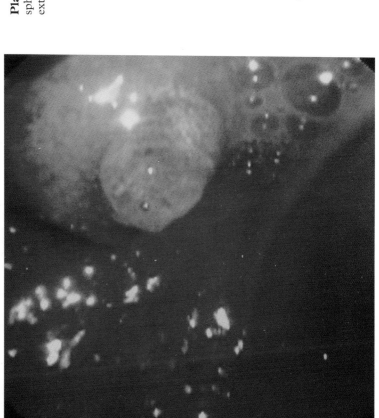

Plate 7 Endoscopic photo of sphincterotomy and stone extraction: Normal papilla.

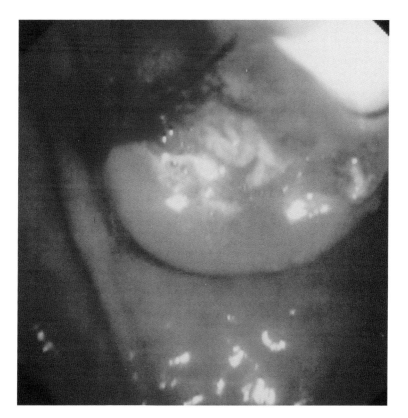

Plate 8 Endoscopic photo of sphincterotomy and stone extraction: A sphincterotome is in position at the papilla and diathermy across the cutting wire divides the sphincter of Oddi.

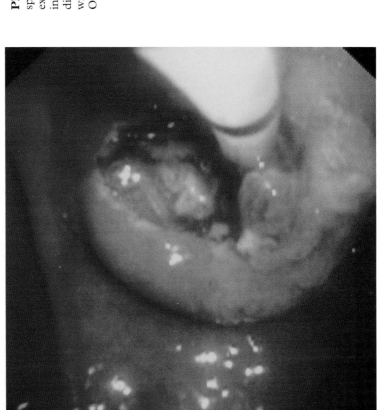

Plate 9 Endoscopic photo of sphincterotomy and stone extraction: a sphincterotome is in position at the papilla and diathermy across the cutting wire divides the sphincter of Oddi.

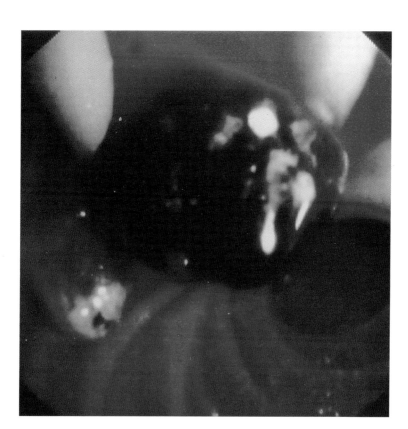

Plate 10 Endoscopic photo of sphincterotomy and stone extraction: stone is extracted with a balloon.

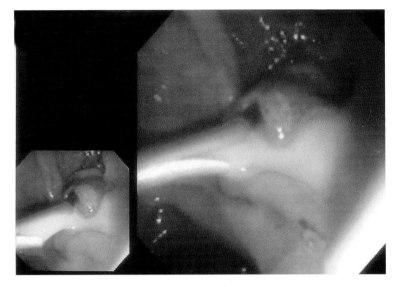

Plate 11 This shows purulent bile exuding from the drainage holes of a new plastic stent inserted across a malignant stricture in a patient who presented with cholangitis.

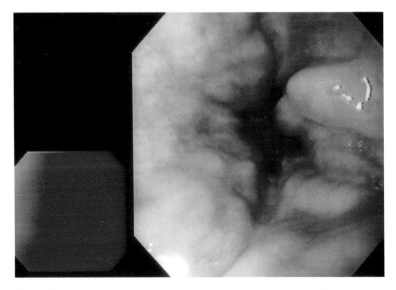

Plate 12 Moderate sized oesophageal varices occupying ¹/₂ of lumen.

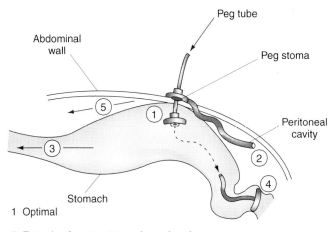

1 Optimal

2 Extrusion from tract to peritoneal cavity

3 Aspiration

4 Migration → intestinal obstruction

5 Local sepsis & cellulitis

Figure 10.1 Complications of PEG.

PEG tube displacement or migration

Clinical features

Migration of a PEG tube to cause gastric outlet obstruction has been reported in 0·9% of cases, usually associated with Foley catheters. Occasional migration to the jejunum and terminal ileum and even one case of obstructive jaundice has been reported due to ampullary obstruction.

In obstructive cases the patient will vomit profusely and rapidly lose weight. Abdominal pain, distension and ileus will be present if obstruction is prolonged.

Management

- The tube must be withdrawn back to its original position or replaced.
- Secure fixation to the abdominal wall will always correct migration.
- Daily observation of the external markings on the tube are necessary if migration is a recurrent problem.

Necrotising fasciitis

Clinical features

This is a dreaded but, fortunately, rare complication of PEG placement. It is a serious, rapidly progressive condition leading to widespread necrosis of the anterior abdominal wall due to a combination of aerobic and anaerobic organisms.

Early signs are erythema around the stoma, with subcutaneous crepitus and the appearance of epidermal bullae. Gas may be seen in the subcutaneous tissues on plain x ray films. Patients may rapidly develop septic shock with a mortality of greater than 38%.

Management

- Remove the PEG tube.
- Arrange a surgical consult – early debridement may be necessary.
- IV fluids and broad spectrum antibiotics.

Further reading

1 Foutch PG. Complications of percutaneous endoscopic gastrostomy and jejunostomy. *Gastrointest Endoscop Clin N Am* 1992;2:231–48.

11 Variceal sclerotherapy, ligation and balloon tamponade

Introduction

The treatment of bleeding oesophageal varices is discussed in Chapter 27. The gastroenterologist has numerous methods available to control variceal haemorrhage such as sclerotherapy, variceal ligation and balloon tamponade. Several prospective randomised studies have demonstrated a lower incidence of complications with variceal ligation compared to sclerotherapy.

The complication of each procedure is discussed in turn.

Complications of balloon tamponade

Balloon tamponade stops acute variceal bleeding in 60–90%. Haemostasis is temporary and definitive treatment needs to be done within 12 h. Complications occur in 10–30%. See Table 11.1

Aspiration pneumonia

Clinical features

Aspiration usually occurs during insertion of the tube. This is a frequent cause of death associated with balloon tamponade.

Management

- Arrange full blood picture, blood cultures, sputum for organisms and sensitivity, chest *x* ray.
- Broad spectrum antibiotics: – cefotaxime 2 g tid iv plus metronidazole 500 mg tid iv.
- Oxygen administration.
- Chest physiotherapy.
- If patient is hypoxic, consider ventilatory support.

Table 11.1 Complications of balloon tamponade.

Complications	Incidence
Aspiration pneumonia	Common
Pressure induced ulceration	Common
Airway obstruction	Rare
Impaction of device	Rare
Oesophageal perforation	Rare

NB: Common < 30%, rare < 2%.

Airway obstruction

Clinical features

This is an acute, life threatening complication that occurs when the gastric balloon deflates, permitting the still inflated oesophageal balloon to migrate proximally and obstruct the upper airway. It occurs more frequently when "active" traction is employed. Endotracheal intubation and mechanical ventilation will reduce the risk.

Management

The tube should be cut using scissors to deflate the balloon and permit rapid removal of the device.

Pressure induced ulceration

Clinical features

In most cases, only inflate the gastric balloon first. If this does not control the bleeding then inflate the oesophageal balloon. Excessive balloon pressure or prolonged use can lead to pressure induced ulceration and necrosis of the oesophageal mucosa. To avoid this, the oesophageal balloon should not be inflated for more than 24 h, with periodic deflation every 6–8 hs. It is essential to monitor the balloon inflation pressures on a regular basis.

Management

- Proton pump inhibitors and sucralfate.
- If this is complicated by bleeding or perforation, see the sections below.

Oesophageal perforation

Clinical features

This is a life threatening complication which occurs in 3% of cases. The oesophagus is the most common site of perforation. It occurs as a consequence of inflation of the gastric balloon within the oesophagus. The risk of perforation may be higher following recent sclerotherapy. Other reported sites include the duodenum and jejunum.

The exact site of the tube should be determined before full inflation is attempted. Tube position can be ascertained by abdominal and chest *x* rays.

Management

- If perforation is suspected, chest *x* ray may show air in the mediastinum. If perforation is more distal to the oesophagus, abdominal *x* ray may show air under the diaphragm.
- Gastrograffin swallow.
- A decision should be made to manage the patient either conservatively or with surgery based on the size of the perforation which can be assessed by gastrograffin swallow and patient's clinical status (see section on oesophageal perforation below).

Impaction

Clinical features

There have been several reports of an inability to remove the tube because of failure to deflate the balloon.

Management

- Do not attempt to forcibly remove the balloon as it can lead to serious injury.
- Endoscopic deflation of the balloon by puncturing it with biopsy forceps or a sclerotherapy needle.
- If this fails, surgery through a combined thoracoabdominal approach may be required.

Complications of endoscopic sclerotherapy

The incidence of serious complications of sclerotherapy ranges from 10 to 20% with a mortality of 0–13%. The most frequent serious complication is bleeding from oesophageal ulcers. The other major complications are oesophageal perforation, mediastinitis and oesophageal stricture. Table 11.2 shows the comprehensive list of documented complications. Only the frequent and serious complications are discussed.

GASTROINTESTINAL EMERGENCIES

Table 11.2 Complications of endoscopic sclerotherapy. There are numerous rare complications which are not mentioned here.

Complications	Incidence
Minor complications	
Superficial oesophageal ulceration	69–94%
Dysphagia/odynophagia	30–70%
Chest pain	30–64%
Fever	20–50%
Major complications	
Oesophageal	
Dysmotility	Common
Stricture (asymptomatic)	4–60%
Stricture (symptomatic)	4–33%
Delayed haemorrhage from ulcer	2–15%
Deep ulceration	Occasional
Gastroesophageal reflux	Occasional
Perforation	0–6%
Pulmonary	
Pleural effusion	Up to 50%
Aspiration pneumonia	Occasional
Atelactasis	Occasional
Bronchitis	Occasional
Vascular	
Congestive gastropathy	Occasional
Ectopic varices	Occasional
Mediastinum	
Mediastinitis	Rare
Infectious	
Bacteraemia	Up to 53%, usually < 10
Bacterial peritonitis	Occasional
Miscellaneous	
Acute renal failure	Occasional

Pain

Clinical features

Substernal pain is noted in about 30–64% and is usually transient, resolving in 6–12 h. Severe pleuritic type pain should be thoroughly investigated with a chest x ray and Gastromiro swallow to rule out perforation.

Management

Adequate analgesia; opiates may be required in 10%.

58

Dysphagia

Clinical features

This is a transient common symptom due to oedema at the injection site. It begins to improve after the first 12–24 h. Dysphagia that develops as a late sequela of sclerotherapy indicates an oesophageal stricture.

Management

- If dysphagia is early, patients should be given liquid diet for first 24–48 h.
- If dysphagia is severe or persistent, endoscopy is indicated. If there is a stricture, it can be dilated safely even if varices are present. A relative contraindication would be presence of large oesophageal ulcers.

Ulcers

Clinical features

Superficial ulcers are commonly seen and may predict a good outcome.

Management

Proton pump inhibitors are effective in healing ulcers.

Bleeding

Clinical features

Post-sclerotherapy bleeding may be:

- Immediate – due to puncture of the varix by the needle.
- Early – bleeding usually occurs within the first 24 h and may result from incomplete sclerotherapy and/or bleeding from remaining varices. Unusually, there may be intramural bleeding with dissection of the oesophageal mucosa resulting in a haematoma (retrosternal pain, dysphagia or odynoophagia).
- Late – due to oesophageal ulcers. Generally occurs within 2 months. Bleeding may involve arterial rupture and may be severe.

Management

- Immediate bleeding – risk is less if the external diameter of the needle is < 0·6 mm. If it happens, sclerosant should be injected above and below the bleeding point. Alternatives include using band ligation of the varices or thrombin glue injection.

- Early and late bleeding – sucralfate may stop rebleeding from sclerotherapy induced ulcers. Propranolol or octreotide may reduce rebleeding rate. Endoscopy is indicated to diagnose and treat the cause of rebleeding. If the cause are varices, band ligation is recommended. Alternatives include repeat sclerotherapy or thrombin glue injection. If rebleeding originates from a deep oesophageal ulcer, it is unwise to perform further sclerotherapy into the ulcer. Options include injecting into the variceal column above and below the bleeding point, using laser or heater probe therapy.

Perforation

Clinical features

Perforation is due to trauma at the time of endoscopy and presentation may be delayed. The high risk period for perforation is within the first 2 weeks. The clinical manifestations of perforation may not be recognised for up to 7 weeks. The presentation includes chest pain, fever, pleural effusion or worsening encephalopathy. Symptoms and signs may be minimal. Mediastinitis usually occurs. Death frequently results (see Chapter18).

Management

- Gastrograffin swallow to demonstrate a leak.
- Conservative management should be tried initially with:
  - nil by mouth
  - gastric suction
  - broad spectrum antibiotics, e.g. cefotaxime 2 g tid iv plus metronidazole 400 mg tid iv
  - total parenteral nutrition
  - intravenous proton pump inhibitors – omeprazole 40 mg iv or pantroprazole 40 mg iv.
- Chest drain should be inserted for a pleural effusion or empyema.
- A surgical consult should be obtained.
- If conservative management fails after 24–48 h, surgery is indicated.

Fever

Clinical features

Fever is common after sclerotherapy occurring in 20–50%. It is usually low grade and lasts only 24–48 h.

Management

- Antibiotic therapy is not required.
- If a fever is high and spiking, persists beyond 48 h or is associated with other evidence of infection, consider sepsis or oesophageal perforation.
- Urgent investigations: full blood picture, blood cultures and chest *x* ray are then indicated.

Pleural effusion

Clinical features

Pleural effusions occur in up to 50% of cases, following sclerotherapy. They are usually exudative in character and small. Uncomplicated effusions spontaneously resolve within days to weeks.

Management

- Uncomplicated pleural effusions require no treatment.
- Presence of high fever, prolonged chest pain, respiratory distress require urgent investigation to rule out empyema or an oesophageal perforation with:
  - full blood picture
  - blood cultures
  - pleural aspiration for appearance of aspirate (purulent indicates empyema or perforation), direct microscopy for white cells and culture
  - gastrograffin swallow to demonstrate or rule out oesophageal perforation.

Complications of endoscopic variceal band ligation

The principle of endoscopic variceal band ligation is similar to that of band ligation of haemorrhoids. An oesophageal varix is sucked into a cylinder attached to the end of an endoscope. A band is then triggered by a wire through the biopsy channel and ligates the base of the varix. The strangulated varix then sloughs off within 2–4 days leaving a shallow ulcer which results in fibrosis and obliteration of the varix. Complications occur in 2–15%. Randomised trials have shown that this is lower than that from sclerotherapy. Most of the complications described in earier series occur as a result of using the overtube. With multiple band ligators now currently being used instead of the single band devices, overtubes are not used and hopefully the overtube related complications should now not be seen. See Table 11.3.

Oesophageal ulceration

Clinical features

Early ulceration occurs in almost all patients. These tend to be shallow and rarely lead to complications. There have been case reports of oesophageal necrosis and perforation.

Management

- Proton pump inhibitors should be routinely given.
- Complications such as bleeding and perforation should be managed as for sclerotherapy complications.

Dysphagia

Clinical features

This is uncommon and has been reported in a case report.

Management

Limit postligation diet to liquids or soft foods for the first 24 h.

Perforation

Clinical features

This is the most serious complication. It is directly related to the use of the overtube which is now not used.

Management

As for perforation following sclerotherapy.

Ectopic and gastric varices

Clinical features

This is the development of ectopic, non-oesophageal, portosystemic varices. A few studies have described a higher incidence of

Table 11.3 Complications of endoscopic variceal band ligation.

Complications	Incidence
Complicated oesophageal ulcer	Rare
Dysphagia	Rare
Ectopic varices	May be more common than with sclerotherapy

this complication with band ligation compared to sclerotherapy. Ectopic varices can form in a variety of anatomic locations and may cause gastrointestinal bleeding of obscure origin. They may occur in the duodenum, jejunum, ileum or rectum.

Management

- Diagnosis may be difficult. Diagnostic modalities depend on mode of presentation, e.g. if small bowel varices are suspected, then enteroscopy may be indicated. Three vessel angiography may detect ectopic varices.
- Treatment options may include transjugular intrahepatic portosystemic shunt (TIPS).

Further reading

1 D'Amico G, Pagliaro L, Bosch J. The treatment of protal hypertension: a meta-analytic review. *Hepatology* 1995;**22**:332–54.
2 Gimson A, Polson R, Westaby D, *et al*. Omeprazole in the management of intractable oesophageal ulceration following injection sclerotherapy. *Gastroenterology* 1990;**99**:1829–31.
3 Johnson PA, Campbell DR, Antonson CW, *et al*.Complications associated with endoscopic band ligation of esophageal varices. *Gastrointest Endosc* 1993;**39**:181–5.
4 Lee J, Liberman D. Complications related to endoscopic haemostasis techniques. *Gastrointest Endosc Clin N Am* 1996;305–21.
5 McKee RF, Garden OJ, Carter DC. Injection sclerotherapy for bleeding varices: risk factors and complications. *Br J Surg* 1991;**78**:1098–101.
6 Vlavianos P, Gimson AES, Westaby D, *et al*. Balloon tamponade in variceal bleeding: use and misuse. *Br Med J* 1989;**298**:1158.
7 Wong RCK, Van Dam J. Complications of balloon tamponade, sclerotherapy, endoscopic variceal ligation, and transjugular intrahepatic portosystemic shunts (TIPS). In Taylor MB, ed. *Gastrointestinal emergencies*, 2nd edn. Baltimore: Williams & Wilkins, 1997: 925–43.

12 ERCP

Introduction

Endoscopic retrograde cholangiopancreatography (ERCP) involves passage of a side-viewing duodenoscope from the mouth to the papilla of Vater and injection of contrast into the pancreatic and/or biliary systems. Therapeutic applications include endoscopic sphincterotomy for stone extraction or sphincter of Oddi dysfunction, balloon dilatation, stenting of strictures and local treatment of pseudocysts.

As there are complications associated with ERCP, the benefits of performing the procedure weighed against other methods of diagnosis and management should outweigh the risk of complications.

Definition

A complication is defined as an undesired event that necessitates management by a doctor after the procedure is completed and requires hospital care, either unplanned admission or prolongation of a planned stay.

Complications

General risks of ERCP are broadly similar to those of upper GI endoscopy (see previous chapter). Table 12.1 shows the specific complications of ERCP. Overall, diagnostic ERCP carries a complication rate of 1–3% with a mortality rate of 0·1–0·2%. Therapeutic ERCP carries a complication rate of approximately 10% and mortality rates of 1%.

Table 12.1 Specific Complications of ERCP.

	Incidence	Mortality
Pancreatitis	1–5% for diagnostic ERCP 7% after sphincterotomy	<0·5%
Bleeding	2%	0·1%
Perforation after sphincterotomy	1%	20%
Basket impaction	?0·4%	0%
Cholangitis	0·9%	0·05%
Cholecystitis	0·5%	<0·1%

Pancreatitis

Clinical features

Post – ERCP pancreatitis is defined as abdominal pain and tenderness with a rise of amylase at least three times normal at more than 24 h after the procedure and without other cause such as perforation.

Severity is defined as:

- mild – hospital stay less than 3 days
- moderate – hospital stay between 4–10 days.
- severe – hospital stay greater than 10 days, development of local complications (e.g. pseudocyst, necrosis), surgery required, intensive care admission and organ dysfunction.

Management

- The management of pancreatitis from ERCP is the same as that of pancreatitis from other causes (see Chapter 23).
- When sphincterotomy has been performed, it is important to rule out retroduodenal perforation as an alternative or accompanying cause of pain. Plain abdominal *x* rays may show retroperitoneal air. If they are negative a CT abdomen may be helpful to rule out perforation and confirm pancreatic oedema.

Bleeding

Clinical features:

This is a potential complication of sphincterotomy. Bleeding is defined as clinical evidence of bleeding (haematemesis and/or melaena) with tachycardia, hypotension or symptoms.

Severity is defined as:

- mild – haemoglobin drop of < 3 g/dl and no need for transfusion,
- moderate – transfusion of four units or less with no angiographic intervention or surgery
- severe – transfusion of five units or more, or intervention (angiographic or surgical) or admission to intensive care unit.

Bleeding can occur less than 24 h (17%) or greater than 24 h (79%) after the procedure.

Management

- Most bleeding stops spontaneously and patients can be managed conservatively.
- Invasive procedures should be considered if the patient does not stop bleeding or rebleeds.
- Endoscopic therapies include injection of adrenaline or application of a bipolar probe.
- Surgery may be required in approximately 25%. This usually consists of oversewing the sphincterotomy with consideration of direct ligation of the gastroduodenal or retroduodenal artery to reduce the risk of rebleeding.
- Angiographic embolisation may be effective but data are limited.

Perforation after sphincterotomy

Clinical features:

Either during the procedure or within a few hours, the patient develops pain, tenderness and fever. Retroperitoneal air may be evident on an abdominal *x* ray. Subcutaneous emphysema, pneumothorax or pneumomediastinum may occur. Portal vein gas may rarely occur.

Small retroperitoneal perforations may be asymptomatic and may be difficult to detect with the clinical presentation resembling acute pancreatitis.

Early CT may show retroperitoneal perforation.

Management

- Surgical consult should be obtained.
- Most patients can be treated conservatively.
- Patients should be put on:
  - nil by mouth
  - nasogastric suction
  - antibiotics: cefotaxime 2 g tid plus metronidazole 400 mg tid iv *or* ciprofloxacin iv

II COMPLICATIONS OF GASTROINTESTINAL PROCEDURES

- proton pump inhibitors – omeprazole 40 mg once daily iv or pantoprazole 40 mg once daily iv.
- Surgical intervention may be necessary in approximately one-third of cases. Failure to improve over a reasonable time frame (24–48 h) or deterioration despite conservative therapy mandates surgery. Early surgery is indicated if the bile duct is still obstructed, e.g. with stones.
- Sealing of the perforation can be revealed by means of CT scan or Gastrograffin swallow.
- Development of a retroperitoneal abscess will require either surgery or percutaneous drainage.

Basket impaction

Clinical features

This can occur if an attempt is made to extract a large stone through a sphincterotomy that is too small or it impacts in a narrowed distal portion of the bile duct.

Management

- Surgery is usually not required.
- Devices such as an external mechanical lithotriptor can be applied to crush the stone or one of the basket wires ruptures.

Cholangitis

Clinical features

Patients can develop cholangitis if an obstructed duct is not drained adequately at the time of ERCP. It can occur following any manipulation of the biliary tree when bile is infected. Symptoms include fever, rigors, jaundice, abdominal pain.

Management

- Appropriate antibiotics such as:
  - Cefotaxime 2 g tid iv plus metronidazole 400 mg tid iv or
  - Ciprofloxacin 400 mg bd iv or 500 mg bd oral
  - Co-amoxiclav 1g qid iv
- If the obstruction persists (e.g. retained stone) or cholangitis does not settle with conservative treatment, urgent repeat ERCP to obtain adequate drainage either with sphincterotomy, extraction of retained stone or biliary stenting should be considered.

Cholecystitis

Clinical features

See Chapter 24 for clinical presentation. Cholecystitis can occur following endoscopic manipulation of the biliary tree, especially in the presence of stones.

Management

- Patients are managed as for acute cholecystitis (see Chapter 24).

Further reading

1 Cotton PB, Lehman G, Vennes J, *et al.* Endoscopic sphincterotomy complications and their management: an attempt at consensus. *Gastrointest Endosc* 1991;**37**:383–93.
2 Freeman M, Nelson D, Sherman S, *et al.* Complications of endoscopic biliary sphincterotomy. *N Engl J Med* 1996;**335**:909–18.
3 Martin D, Tweedle D. Retroperitoneal perforation during ERCP and endoscopic sphincterotomy: causes, clinical features and management. *Endoscopy* 1990;**22**:174–5.
4 Safrany L. Endoscopic treatment of biliary tract disease. *Lancet* 1978;**2**:983–5.
5 Shields S, Carr-Locke DL. Sphincterotomy techniques and risks. *Gastrointest Endosc Clin N Am* 1996;**6**:17–42.
6 Vandervoort J, Tham TCK, Roston A, *et al.* Prospective analysis of risk factors for pancreatitis after diagnostic and therapeutic ERCP. *Gastrointest Endosc* 1996;**43**:400.

13 Laparoscopic cholecystectomy

Introduction

Laparoscopic cholecystectomy is the procedure of choice for the majority of patients with symptomatic gallstones. Advantages of the laparoscopic approach compared to open cholecystectomy include less postoperative pain, shorter hospital stay and quicker recovery time.

Complications

Laparoscopic cholecystectomy is associated with a 2–8% complication rate and mortality of 0–0·5% which compares favourably with open cholecystectomy. See Tables 13.1 and 13.2.

Biliary injuries

The incidence of reported iatrogenic biliary tract injuries during laparoscopic cholecystectomy ranges from 0 to 1% compared to 0·1–0·2% during open cholecystectomy. Classification of bile duct injuries is shown in Table 13.3.

Clinical features

The time period for clinical presentation and recognition of bile duct injuries is highly variable and dependent on the nature of the injury.

A bile leak usually presents early. The mean period to postoperative detection is 8 days. The patient may complain of severe, diffuse abdominal pain, nausea, bloating and fatigue. There may be a low grade pyrexia, mild leukocytosis.

Biliary strictures usually present later; as long as 3 months after cholecystectomy. They may present with jaundice, cholangitis, elevated liver enzymes or abdominal pain.

Table 13.1 Laparoscopic injuries during laparoscopic cholecystectomies: a US survey of 77 604 cases (from Deziel *et al.*, 1993).

Injury Site	No. of patients (%)
Bile ducts	
Common bile duct	271
Common hepatic duct	38
Right hepatic duct	8
Aberrant hepatic duct	48
Cystic duct	94
Total	458 (0·59)
Retroperitoneal vessels	
Aorta	13
Inferior vena cava	5
Iliac artery	11
Iliac vein	7
Total	36 (0·05)
Portal vessels	
Hepatic artery	44
Cystic artery	73
Portal vein	5
Total	122 (0·16)
Other intraabdominal vessels	35 (0·05)
Total vascular	193 (0·25)
Bowel	
Small intestine	57
Colon	35
Duodenum	12
Stomach	5
Total	109 (0·14)

Management

- Morbidity and mortality are minimised when successful management of bile duct injuries is accomplished early.
- Abdominal ultrasound or CT assesses whether or not there is extrahepatic biliary obstruction and the presence or absence of bile collections.
- If a bile collection is found in the right upper quadrant, it should be drained percutaneously.
- If a leak or obstruction is present, an ERCP should be undertaken to define the site and extent of the biliary injury with endoscopic therapy if indicated. An exception may be the situation where bile drainage through the drain decreases suggesting healing of the leak and no further intervention may be required.

Table 13.2 Causes of death after laparoscopic cholecystectomy: a US study of 77 604 cases (from Deziel *et al.*, 1993).

Causes of death	No. of patients (%)
Operative injury	
Bile duct	5
Aorta	3
Small intestine	2
Colon	2
Gallbladder bed bleed	2
Hepatic artery	1
Portal vein	1
Cystic duct leak/sepsis	1
Duodenum	1
Total	18 (0·02)
Non-technical	
Myocardial infarction	3
Pulmonary embolism	3
Pneumonia	2
Ischaemic bowel	2
Respiratory failure	1
Necrotizing fasciitis	1
AIDS/sepsis	1
Unknown	2
Total	15 (0·02)

- The most common is leakage from the cystic duct stump (type A) followed by junction of the cystic duct with the bile duct (type D) and duct of Luschka (type A).
- Leaks can be treated by endoscopic stent placement or sphincterotomy. If there are associated common bile duct stones, they should be removed following a sphincterotomy. Complete bile

Table 13.3 Classification of bile duct injuries.

	Type of injury
Type A	Bile leaks from the cystic duct and ducts of Luschka (from right hepatic lobe in the gallbladder fossa to right hepatic or common bile duct)
Type B	Occlusion of aberrant right hepatic duct
Type C	Leakage of right hepatic duct
Type D	Lateral trauma to the main bile duct causing leakage
Type E	Involves common and main hepatic ducts and correspond to Bismuth classification types I–V

duct occlusion from a clip or ligature precludes endoscopic therapy. Type E is most severe and requires expert management by a hepatobiliary team. A Roux-en-Y hepaticojejunostomy is the procedure of choice for complete ductal transection or for high grade stricture.

Bleeding

Clinical features

Uncontrolled bleeding during laparoscopic cholecystectomy occurs in 0·3 to 0·6% of procedures. Delayed bleeding in the early postoperative period (during the first 48 h) may occur from displaced cystic artery clips or from incompletely electrocoagulated arterial bleeding points Late vascular injuries such as hepatic artery pseudoaneurysms, may result in haemobilia.

Management

- The two most common sites of intraoperative bleeding include the bed of the gallbladder and a posterior branch of the cystic artery. Irrigation is used for precise identification of the bleeding site followed by haemostasis.
- If delayed bleeding occurs, reoperation either open or laparoscopic, is required to control the bleeding.

Bowel injury

Clinical features

The incidence of bowel injury may occur during insertion of the Veress needle or trocars. It may occur due to unrecognised thermal injury to the duodenum resulting in full-thickness necrosis with subsequent perforation. The clinical presentation is typically delayed several days later.

Management

- Similar to that for a perforated duodenal ulcer (see Chapter 20).

Infection

Clinical features

Spillage of gallstones into the peritoneal cavity occurs commonly during laparoscopic cholecystectomy.

Management

- Retrieval of these spilled stones is recommended to prevent the possibility of later subhepatic, subphrenic, intraabdominal,

pelvic, or cutaneous abscess formation, sinus or fistula formation, bowel obstruction or perforation.
- When complete retrieval of the stones is impossible, the right
  subphrenic and subhepatic spaces should be thoroughly irri-
  gated.
- If intraperitoneal stones are identified postoperatively, a
  laparotomy is not warranted.

Pneumoperitoneum

Clinical features

Presents in the initial 24 h after the operation. Patients complain
of shoulder pain referred from diaphragmatic "irritation" from the
pressurised pneumoperitoneum. A pneumothorax may present
with shortness of breath.

Management

- The shoulder pain is rarely severe and resolves spontaneously.
- Chest x ray should be performed if the patient is short of
  breath. A pneumothorax may be treated with observation if
  small and mildly symptomatic. If it is large and symptomatic,
  a chest drain or aspiration may be required.

Retained common bile duct stones

Clinical features

Such stones can present as cholangitis, bile leak, jaundice, pancreatitis, or recurrent biliary colic.

Management

ERCP should be performed and if stones are found, removed
following sphincterotomy.

Further reading

1 Bjorkman DJ, Carr-Locke DL, Lichtenstein DR, *et al.* Post-surgical bile leaks: a short
   transpapillary stent is enough. *Am J Gastroenterol* 1995;**90**:2128–33.
2 Deziel DJ, *et al.* Complications of laparoscopic cholecystectomy: a national survey of 4 292
   hospitals and an analysis of 77 604 cases. *Am J Surg* 1993;**165**:9–14.
3 Madariago JR, Dodson SF, Selby R, Todo S, Iwatsuki S, Starzl TE. Corrective treatment and
   anatomic considerations for laparoscopic cholecystectomy injuries. *J Am Coll Surg* 1994;
   179:321–5.
4 Melin MM, Kollmorgen CF, Sarr MG. Complications of intraabdominal laparoscopic
   surgery. In: Taylor MD, ed. *Gastrointestinal emergencies*, 2nd edn. Baltimore: Williams &
   Wilkins, 1997: 969–80.
5 Southern Surgeons Club. A prospective analysis of 1518 laparoscopic cholecystectomies. *N
   Engl J Med* 1991;**324**:1073–8.

14 Liver biopsy

Introduction

Certain groups of patient are at risk of complications. Relative contraindications are:

- right side empyema
- right sub-phrenic infections.

Absolute contraindications are:

- ascites
- confused/unco-operative patients
- bleeding disorder – a platelet count less than 100 000 and a PTT >15 s
- lack of blood transfusion support
- echinococcal disease
- possible vascular liver mass.

Despite adequate prior assessment and experienced operators, complication rates have been reported in between 0·9–3·7% of procedures within 2 h of the biopsy. Fatal complications usually occur within 6 h of the procedure.

The main complications of liver biopsy are shown in Table 14.1

Treatment of complications

Pain

Clinical features

Up to 22% of patients will complain of dull right upper quadrant or right shoulder tip pain after biopsy.

Table 14.1 Complications of liver biopsy.

Complication	Incidence %
Pain	0·05–22
Haemorrhage (Hepatic)	0·05–23
Billiary peritonitis	0·03–0·22
Bacteraemia	5·8–13·5
Pneumothorax	0·08–0·28
AV Fistula	5·4
Biopsy of other organs	0·003–0·1
Overall mortality	0·008–0·3

Management

- This should be treated with non-opiate analgesics which may be required for several days.
- Pain which is severe, extending into the abdomen or the chest may indicate bleeding (see below).

Haemorrhage

As the liver is a vascular organ, bleeding is the most serious and life-threatening complication. Bleeding is more common in elderly patients or after multiple passes of the needle.

The various sites for bleeding are shown in Figure 14.1.

Intraperitoneal bleeding

Clinical features:

This is usually seen within 2–3 h. The patient will complain of right-sided abdominal pain and may be shocked.

Management

- Check haemoglobin.
- Alert blood bank and order 4 units of blood.
- Insert iv cannula and start crystalloid infusion.
- Call a surgeon for initial consultation.
- Continued bleeding may require a laparotomy with surgical repair of the bleeding point. If the patient is unfit for surgery, an hepatic arteriogram may display the site of bleeding and direct embolisation can be attempted.

Intra-hepatic haematomas

Clinical features

These are commonly reported on ultra sound scans after biopsy and may be asymptomatic. However, continued pain and a drop in

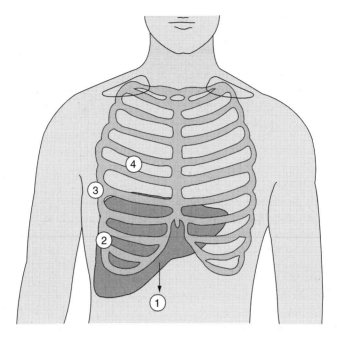

1. Intraperitoneal

2. Liver capsular haematoma

3. Intra-pleural / thoracic

4. Pulmonary → severe haemothorax

Figure 14.1 Potential bleeding sites after percutaneous liver biopsy.

haemoglobin should point to an expanding or sub-capsular haematoma

Management

- Transfuse if necessary as above.
- Ask for surgical opinion.
- Ultra sound to define extent and size as baseline.
- Observe as most settle with conservative therapy.

Haemobilia

Clinical features

This form of bleeding is associated with the classical triad of symptoms:

- gastro-intestinal bleeding – usually melaena
- biliary colic
- jaundice.

The average time after biopsy and onset of symptoms is 5 days. The diagnosis may be assisted by U/S of the biliary tree and ERCP may show blood coming from the ampulla and clot in the CBD on the cholangiogram.

Management

- Coagulation defects should be corrected if present using fresh frozen plasma 6 units, platelet infusion or vitamin K.
- Transfuse with blood as required.
- If bleeding continues – surgery or angiography and embolisation.

Bacteraemia

Clinical features:

This may often occur sub-clinically. If a patient develops abdominal pain and pyrexia within 24 h of biopsy, this complication should be considered.

Management

- Send blood for WBC and differential.
- Blood cultures.
- U/S to rule out liver abscess (rare).
- Start antibiotics – amoxycillin 1 g/6 h plus metronidazole 500 mg/8 h or cefuroxime 750 mg/8 h with metronidazole 500 mg/8 h iv.

Pulmonary Complications

Clinical features

Pleural and pulmonary complications can occur as the biopsy needle traverses the right pleural cavity.

The patient may complain of right sided pleuritic pain, either at the time of biopsy or 2–3 hours later. Rarely haemoptysis or cough occurs.

Management

- Aspirate effusion if it appears to be causing symptoms.

- A chest drain will be necessary if a pneumothorax > 30% of pleural cavity is present.

Further reading

1 Piccinino F, Sagnelli E, Pasquale G, et al. Complications following percutaneous liver biopsy: a multi-centre retrospective study on 68 276 biopsies. *J Hepatol* 1986;2:165–73.

15 Colonoscopy

Introduction

There are two major complications:

- haemorrhage
- perforation.

Complications

Haemorrhage

Clinical features:

This is invariably associated with biopsy or polypectomy. Recent surveys have not shown a relationship between age, sex or polyp size and risk. Haemorrhage may be *immediate* or *delayed*. The former is associated with the use of blended diathermy current, while the latter is associated with the use of pure coagulation current. Cold mucosal biopsy is associated with a higher risk in patients on NSAIDs so it is advisable to stop these drugs 7 days before colonoscopy if possible.

Management of immediate haemorrhage

- If the bleeding spot is identified as a polyp stalk, the remnant should be resnared gently and held for 5 min. If bleeding is seen to recur after slow release of the snare, short bursts of pure coagulation current should be applied.
- Adrenaline 1:10 000 can be injected directly into the bleeding site if the above fails.
- BICAP or heater probe can be used if available, although their use is more hazardous in the right colon and caecum. Argon plasma beamer is also effective for the superficial vessel.
- Should bleeding persist, a mesenteric angiogram will help to

show the vessel(s) involved and vasopressin can be infused locally to effectively vasoconstrict the mucosal feeding arterioles.

Management of delayed haemorrhage

- If the bleeding is active, the patient should be given a routine colonic lavage with polyethylene glycol solution and colonoscopy as soon as possible.
- If the bleeding site is seen, haemostasis should be attempted using the modalities above.
- Mesenteric angiography should be carried out if bleeding recurs.

Perforation

Clinical features

The incidence of this complication ranges from 0–0·9% in large surveys. The commonest sites are recto-sigmoid and sigmoid-descending junction. Perforation is more commonly associated with severe diverticular disease, infammatory bowel disease, radiation colitis and multiple colonic adhesions. The clinical features of perforation are listed below:

- abdominal pain with increasing rigidity
- abdominal distension
- guarding – localised at first then generalised
- loss of liver dullness
- loss of bowel sounds
- inability to insufflate/deflate colon.

Although the presentation may be dramatic, silent perforations can occur or signs may be masked for hours or days by omental plugging. If in doubt a plain abdominal *x* ray or CT scan should be obtained.

Management

- Early surgery is indicated if:
  - peritoneal signs develop in 4–6 h
  - there are signs of systemic sepsis or the patient's condition deteriorates clinically
  - there is distal colonic obstruction.

All patients, after the diagnosis is suspected, should be given iv antibiotics to cover Gram Positive and Gram Negative organisms.

- Adequate pain relief with iv pethidine 50–100 mg is necessary.
- *Conservative management* has been advocated.
  - when a small perforation occurs in asymptomatic patients,
  - if the perforation is localised after 6-8 h
  - patient has no systemic symptoms.

In these situations the patient must be closely observed in hospital while fasting on iv fluids and antiobiotic cover.

- In all cases an early surgical consultation should be obtained so that the subsequent management plan can be devised.

Rare complications of colonoscopy – pneumatosis coli, subcutaneous emphysema

Clinical features

Occasionally insufflated gas can pass into the retroperitoneum, bowel wall (pneumatosis coli), or subcutaneous tissues leading to abdominal discomfort and signs of subcutaneous emphysema.

Management

- In these situations, a perforation into the peritoneal cavity with septic risk must be excluded as described above.
- If the patient has no signs of peritoneal inflammation or of systemic sepsis, a conservative approach can safely be employed although it is advisable to monitor the patient in hospital and obtain an urgent surgical consult.

Part III
Specific conditions

16 Foreign body impaction in the oesophagus

Introduction

Foreign body impaction in the oesophagus is associated with significant morbidity and mortality which is usually due to perforation and subsequent sepsis. This emergency is encountered more frequently in children but adults make up 20% of cases. Adult risk factors include alcohol and drug abuse, mental illness and the wearing of dentures. Food impaction is associated with concomitant oesophageal disease, usually gastro-oesophageal reflux. Recurrent episodes of impaction always suggest the presence of an oesophageal stricture. Seventy per cent of impaction occurs in the cervical region, 20% in the mid oesophagus and 10% in the distal part.

History and examination

Most patients give a history of recent dysphagia or something "sticking in the throat". Odynophagia may be present. Some patients will recall the object ingested. Chest pain, salivation and regurgitation may be present and the latter two symptoms point to complete oesophageal obstruction. Severe chest pain suggests oesophageal perforation. Respiratory obstruction will be present in 5% of cases due to impaction in the cervical region.

Treatment

The management of this emergency is summarised in Figure 16.1. The main steps in management are:

1   Immediate evaluation of the airway

muscle at 15–17 cm from the incisor teeth is a common site of impaction in the upper oesophagus. The aortic arch and the left main bronchus compress the mid oesophagus, while the lower oesophagus proximal to the hiatus at 36–38 cm is a site commonly associated with peptic strictures and carcinoma.

- The timing of endoscopy – the optimum times to plan endoscopic retrieval are shown in Table 16.1. The time after 24 h from initial impaction has been associated with a higher rate of complications. Endoscopy time depends on the type of object obstructing, the site of obstruction and whether obstruction is thought to be complete or partial.
- Endoscopy should only be attempted when the full range of retrieval accessories are on hand:
  - alligator forceps
  - rat-tooth forceps
  - dormier baskets
  - polyp retrieval snares
  - overtube – for sharp objects.

Endoscopic removal of specific foreign bodies

The most important factor prior to endoscopy is to secure a safe airway. If airway patency is in doubt or the oesophagus is likely to be full of debris, general anaesthesia is essential.

Coins

- Larger coins such as the 50 pence or US quarter lodge at the cricopharyngeus and are shown on *x* ray films.
- After endoscopic intubation,the coin is visualised and grasped with alligator-type forceps. The scope should be withdrawn straight with the patient in Trendelenberg position.
- If a coin passes into the stomach, extraction is rarely necessary.

Table 16.1 (After Webb WA, Taylor MB. 1997).

Foreign body	Location	Time endoscopy(h)
Coin	Upper	4–6
Coin	Lower	12–18
Meat	Any/complete obs	Urgent
Meat	Any/incomplete obs	8–10
Sharps	Any	4–6

Food bolus impaction

- This is the most common cause of this emergency situation in adults.
- Impaction is likely to involve the distal oesophagus.
- If the patient cannot swallow saliva, complete obstruction is likely and emergency endoscopy is indicated to reduce the risk of aspiration.
- If the obstruction is incomplete, the bolus may pass with time and endoscopic removal is less urgent.
- A soft food bolus can be removed in its entirety with polyp removal snare.
- As the bolus is withdrawn up the oesophagus within the snare, it should be pulled close to the endoscope tip as it passes through the relatively narrower cricopharyngeal region to avoid dislodgement.
- Large boluses may be removed piecemeal. If a piecemeal approach is used, the prior passage of an overtube will avoid discomfort to the patient from repeated intubations.
- In some cases of soft food bolus impaction, a "push" technique can be used. If there is no distal obstruction, the bolus can be gently forced downwards into the stomach. As the oesophago-gastric junction turns to the left at the hiatus, it is important to direct the push from the right side. When the bolus has been cleared, the lower oesophagus should be inspected for strictures which can be managed accordingly.

Sharp foreign objects

- These are the most hazardous to deal with due to the risk of trauma on retreival. Needles, bones, dental bridgework and even razor blades may be encountered.
- It is safer to use an overtube in these patients.
- The object should be grasped so that the sharp end is "trailing" on withdrawal. The object can be pulled inside the overtube at the level of retrieval, when it can be removed safely with the endoscope.

Button batteries

- Ingestion of these objects from pocket calculators, watches and hearing aids is a growing problem, especially in children.
- If impaction occurs, the chemical contents may react with the

oesophageal mucosa causing pressure necrosis or localised chemical or low voltage burns

- A history of battery ingestion should be confirmed with a chest *x* ray followed by urgent endoscopic retrieval with either a Dormier basket or a balloon retrieval catheter.

Further reading

1 Crysdale W, Sendi K, Yoo J. Esophageal foreign bodies in children. *Ann Otol Rhino Laryngol* 1991;**100**:320–4
2 Webb W. Management of foreign bodies in the upper gastro-intestinal tract: update. *Gastrointest Endosc* 1995;**41**:39–50.

17 Caustic ingestion to the oesophagus

Introduction

The ingestion of caustic substances can result in devastating injuries to the oesophageal mucosa. Alkaline household cleaning products and lye soaps tend to cause more oesophageal damage while strong acids inflict more damage on the stomach. The ingestion of small button batteries, often by young children, also gives rise to alkali damage due to their high concentration of sodium and potassium hydroxide.

Mechanism of injury

Exposure of the squamous epithelium of the oesophagus to strong alkali results in liquefactive necrosis of cells due to saponification of cell membranes and denaturation of cell wall proteins. Damage may extend beyond the oesophageal wall to involve adjacent mediastinal structures. The gastric mucosa may be protected due to acid neutralisation of the ingested alkali but sufficient doses of the latter will result in gastric erosion, perforation and peritonitis. Animal studies have shown that the initial acute phase progresses to sloughing of the necrotic mucosa resulting in ulcers after 5–10 days. Finally, collagenous strictures form at 4–6 weeks.

The ingestion of acid is much less common. The result is coagulation necrosis of the mucosal cells with the production of a firm eschar. The oesophagus may be spared from severe damage in acid ingestion cases.

History and examination

Some substances will cause injury to the oro-pharynx or predominantly to the oesophagus and stomach. Typically oro-pharyngeal damage results in drooling of saliva, sore throat and coughing. Laryngeal oedema causes stridor, hoarseness and aphonia. If the patient has aspirated a quantity of the substance, dyspnoea may be a dominant symptom. Oral pain may be a significant symptom.

Oesophageal mucosal damage results in chest pain, dyshagia and odynophagia within a few hours, while gastric injury results in retching, vomiting and epigastric pain.

Symptoms may settle from days 5–15 until scarring starts in the oesophagus resulting in stricturing and dysphagia for solids then liquids.

Gastric outlet obstruction is an occasional late sequel.

Investigations

- *Plain radiographs* of the chest and abdomen should be obtained to rule out pulmonary aspiration, mediastinal perforation and free abdominal gas.
- Endoscopy should be performed in all patients within 12–24 h *unless* the patient is shocked, has severe oropharyhgeal oedema and necrosis, severe respiratory distress , mediastinal or intra-abdominal free air. An endoscopic grading of caustic mucosal injury has been Kirsh and Ritter (see Table 17.1)

Treatment of caustic ingestions

- *Emesis should not be induced* and the patient should wash out their mouth and gargle with water without swallowing as soon as possible.
- *Signs of airway compromise* mean that life-threatening laryngeal oedema may be present and an anaesthetist should be called to inspect the larynx by indirect laryngoscopy. At this stage it may be necessary to sedate the patient and pass an endotracheal support for ventilatory support.

Table 17.1 Endoscopic grading of caustic injury.

Degree/stage	Endoscopic findings
1	Erythema, oedema
2a	Friablity, bleeding, erosions and ulcers
2b	2a and deep or circumferential ulcers
3a	Necrotic black areas with deep ulcers
3b	Extensive necrosis

- Intravenous fluids are required if the patient is hypotensive.
- It is important to try and establish the type of ingested substance at this stage when the patient is stabilised. A blood toxicology screen should be sent in case a suicidal patient has ingested other drugs e.g. paracetamol, anti-depressants

Endoscopy

- Endoscopy should be performed in all patients within 12–24 h unless the patient is shocked, has severe oropharyhgeal oedema and necrosis, severe respiratory distress, mediastinal or intra-abdominal free air. An endoscopic grading of caustic mucosal injury has been described by Kirsh and Ritter (see Table 17.1)
- Endoscopic findings have very important bearing on prognostic and therapeutic outcome.
- Patients with grade 1 and 2a injuries usually develop no long term complications.
- Patients with grade 2b have up to 70% risk of stricture.
- Grade 3 injuries are associated with the highest rates of long term morbidity. In all grade 3 injuries, 90% develop strictures within the first 8 weeks.
- Grade 3b particularly develop acute complications in 70% of cases and have a mortality rate of 65%.
- Perendoscopic dilatation is usually needed to treat strictures initially but this can later be changed to peroral bougienage which may need to be frequent.

In-hospital management

The recommended management of patients according to mucosal injury grade after endoscopy are shown in Table 17.2.

Steroids

There is no clear evidence to support the routine use of iv steroids in these patients

Antibiotics

These are no longer recommended routinely unless specific septic complications arise

Nasogastric tubes and swallowed strings

Some studies have suggested that the passage of a soft NG feeding tube facilitates later dilatation should strictures occur. However

Table 17.2 Management summary in caustic ingestion.

Injury grade	Treatment
1 (Low risk)	Observe, fluid diet Home 24 h, Barium swallow at 4 weeks
2a (Low risk)	Observe, fluid diet, start oral PPI Watch for early airway compromise Home 24 h, Barium swallow 1 month
2b & 3a (High risk)	Observe in HDU/ICU setting, Start iv PPI, antibiotics, must be fasted for 48 h. Home in 72 h if taking fluid diet. Will require close follow-up to detect stricture formation or gastric outlet obstruction
3b (V. high risk, high mortality)	As for 3a but if signs of oesophageal or gastro- duodenal perforation, surgery may be indicated. Shock, sepsis and tracheo-bronchial injury need to be treated as they arise

opponents of this therapy state that an indwelling tube may actually promote further inflammatory damage.

Stents

There is no clear evidence to suggest that early stenting reduces further late morbidity.

Total parenteral nutrition

There is no good evidence that this form of feeding from an early stage prevents stricture formation but it may be needed as support therapy in stages 2b, 3a and 3b.

Further reading

1 Gumaste VV, Dave PB. Ingestion of corrosive substances by adults. *Am J Gastroenterol* 1992; **87**:1–5.

18 Oesophageal perforation

Introduction

Due to its associated high mortality (10–45%), this is considered one of the most serious gastro-intestinal emergencies requiring a high index of suspicion in some cases if diagnosis is to be made promptly after the event.

Aetiology

The main causes of perforation are outlined below

- Iatrogenic – the commonest cause resulting in 33–75·5% of all cases. The trauma may be due to endoscopic intubation, dilatation, sclerotherapy or laser ablation. Intra-operative perforation can result from anti-reflux surgery, myotomy, pneumonectomy or mediastinoscopy
- Boerhaave's syndrome – accounts for 7–19% of cases. This is spontaneous rupture of the oesophagus during vomiting. Predisposing factors include coughing, childbirth, hyperemesis gravidarum, status asthmaticus, weightlifting and alcohol abuse
- Chest trauma – accounts for 8–15·8% of all cases and may be sharp penetrating or blunt

History

The initial clinical features depend on the site of the injury. In high cervical perforations patients complain of neckpain, dysphonia, dysphagia and hoarseness. Subcutaneous emphysema is an early important sign.

In thoracic perforations, the patient complains of chest pain, dysphagia, and odynophagia.

Examination

Physical signs include:
- cyanosis
- upper abdominal rigidity
- subcutaneous emphysema
- signs of pericardial tamponade may be present.

Investigations

Prompt diagnosis is essential as delay can result in higher rates of sepsis, shock and mortality. The following investigations are useful in suspected cases.
- Lateral radiograph of neck may show air in the prevertebral tissue planes.
- Chest radiograph may demonstrate pneumomediastinum, subcutaneous emphysema, pleural effusion and hydropneumothorax.
- In the absence of signs from the above, Gastrografin contrast studies will usually demonstrate a perforation, although a false negative study will be found in 10%. Barium can also be used as the contrast medium.
- CT can detect small fluid collections and may help to assess the degree of mediastinal involvement.

Management

Treatment options are conservative and surgical. In all cases, early surgical consultation should be obtained and a joint management approach is essential.

Conservative management is indicated in the following conditions
- Absence of respiratory failure, shock or sepsis
- The perforation is well contained in the cervical region or mediastinum and there is no progressive intra-mediastinal or peritoneal involvement
- Absence of distal oesophageal stricture

In all patients treated conservatively:

- Total parenteral nutrition should be commenced.
- Broad spectrum antibiotics should be started and continued for 10–14 days intravenously. The antibiotic choice should cover gram negative organisms and anaerobes. Cefuroxime 750 mg or amoxycillin 1 g plus metronidazole 500 mg/8 h are an appropriate choice.
- Continuous NG suction should be maintained.
- The insertion of an intercostal drain to aspirate a pleural effusion may be necessary.

Surgical management

- If a patient does not meet the above criteria for care or if there is loss of containment of the perforation associated with persistent pain and/or sepsis then operative management appears to be the best treatment option (see Figure 18.1).
- Cervical perforations are best treated conservatively and result in 100% survival.
- The surgical approach to thoracic or intra-abdominal perforations if the diagnosis is made within 24 h is to carry out a

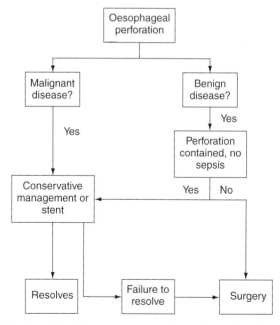

Figure 18.1 Algorithm for management of oesophageal perforation after dilatation/instrumentation.

local drainage and re-inforced primary closure in the absence of distal obstruction.

• The longer diagnosis is delayed, the greater is the potential for local tissue necrosis and infection with anaerobic organisms. In some instances the surgeon may decide to close the gastric cardia and divert the upper oesophagus through an end or side oesophagostomy which can be closed at a later date when sepsis has been completely cleared.

• Oesophageal resection is an option in patients with considerable mediastinal soiling especially in the presence of malignant disease with distal obstruction but it is associated with a high mortality and rarely attempted.

19 Complications of oesophageal cancer

Introduction

The management of oesophageal cancer is mainly palliative as 60% of cases are not resectable at presentation and the 5 year survival is 5–7% for squamous tumours and 9% for adenocarcinomas. During the survival period after palliation, considerable morbidity may be encountered some of which requires acute assessment and management.

Aetiology

The complications which give rise to emergencies are:

- luminal obstruction due to food bolus impaction in a stricture or a stent
- perforation – either spontaneous or iatrogenic due to dilator, stent or laser
- sepsis
- fistulisation
- bleeding
- obstruction due to tumour growth or ingrowth into a stent.

Oesophageal obstruction

Clinical features

In this situation the patient may have been previously diagnosed and received specific therapy for the obstruction with endoscopic dilators, laser ablation or radio/chemotherapy. The progression of dysphagia slowly over several days or weeks will eventually result in complete dysphagia with drooling due to failure to swallow even saliva. When this happens in the absence of a history suggesting food impaction, the patient should be treated as an obstructive emergency due to the high risk of rapid dehydration and pulmonary aspiration.

The patient should be managed as follows:

Management

- The patient should be admitted to hospital.
- IV fluids should be started and the patient kept "nil by mouth".
- Signs of aspiration should be sought.
- A small volume barium swallow radiograph will help to identify the site and length of the stricture. (Barium is less irritant to the lungs than gastrograffin if aspirated). This test will also identify a fistula or early perforation.
- The lesion should then be examined with an endoscope. It is unlikely that even a paediatric endoscope will pass beyond the upper level of the stricture. In new presentations biopsies or cytology brushings can be taken.
- Mercury filled bougies should be avoided and a guide – wire passed under *x* ray control. In tight strictures with complex lumens, a toposcopic, lumen-finding catheter or a "hydrophilic" or "slippery" wire can be very useful in passing the stricture.
- Once the guide-wire is in place, dilatation can be carried out using tapered polyvinyl dilators (Savary) which have largely replaced olive shaped dilators.
- The lumen can be gradually and gently dilated until it can admit an adult-sized endoscope.
- The patient can then be assessed for surgical resection, radiotherapy or the insertion of a prosthesis.

Unfortunately, simple dilatation therapy will result in restricturing in most cases. Radiotherapy will probably delay the need for dilatation but the effect is unpredictable in most cases.

Food impaction obstruction

In this case the patient may present for the first time, usually with a fairly short history of dysphagia. In some cases, oesophageal cancer will have been previously diagnosed and a stent may have been placed (see below). The management of food bolus impaction is discussed in Chapter 16.

Complications of stents

Clinical features

Dilatation alone usually has a short effect in the management of malignant strictures and the placement of a prosthesis or stent in the oesophageal lumen across a stricture is an option for palliation.

Plastic stents had been used. These stents are traumatic and difficult to insert with considerable morbidity. The development of metal self-expanding stents e.g. Wallstent (Schneider, USA) have become popular because they can be placed over a guidewire in a relatively small lumen and the actual insertion technique is less traumatic for the patient. They are more expensive than plastic stents. Studies comparing plastic with metal stents have shown that metal stents are superior as they are associated with fewer procedure related complications and mortality and are much easier to deploy. In most centres, metal stents have superseded plastic stents.

The main complications of metal stents are listed below:

- perforation (see below)
- stent may fail due to poor placement or migration
- oesophageal bleeding (see below)
- pulmonary aspiration
- tumour overgrowth at top or bottom
- food impaction
- reflux oesophagitis
- erosion into mediastinum, bronchus or aorta

Management

- Tumour overgrowth or ingrowth leading to stent occlusion can be identified endoscopically and treated by radiotherapy, laser ablation, injection of chemicals, insertion of another stent within the old stent, bipolar coagulation or argon plasma beam coagulation.
- The stents can be recanalised and may continue to give adequate palliation.
- Food impaction in or above a stent should be prevented if possible by instructing the patient to take small bites of food, chew well and drink fluids with meals. If impaction occurs it should be treated as for stricture impaction.

Perforation

Clinical features

This complication may occur either spontaneously through the cancer into the underlying normal tissues of the mediastinum or, more commonly, following attempts at palliation of the obstruction by dilators, laser or during stent placement. The perforation during dilatation usually occurs in normal tissue proximal to the stricture rather than in the body of the stricture itself.

In laser perforations, the site is usually a direct burn penetrating the tumour and underlying normal oesophageal wall which may be infiltrated.

The clinical signs of acute perforation have been discussed in the relevant chapter and include:

- chest,neck or abdominal pain
- fever
- dyspnoea
- tachycardia
- surgical emphysema
- pleural effusion
- systemic sepsis.

Diagnosis is confirmed by chest radiographs, plain abdominal radiographs or a water-soluble contrast study. The classic signs of pnemomediastinum and sub-diaphragmatic air will suggest the diagnosis in 50% of cases.

Management

Treatment options are limited because these patients are not fit for surgery. The patients should be treated conservatively in all cases with:

- IV fluids and nil by mouth.
- IV antibiotics to cover Gram positive and negative aerobes and anaerobes.
- In some cases, the placement of oesophageal prosthesis may seal the leak and has been reported to be successful in 60–90% of patients.
- In severe cases a surgically placed gastrostomy can be placed for feeding but the outlook for these patients is poor.

Fistula

Clinical features

Fistula between the oesophageal lumen and the mediastinum are found in 5% of oesophageal cancer patients usually associated with squamous cell carcinoma.

Patients with broncho-oesophageal fistula present with a chronic cough, fever, and evidence of aspiration pneumonia. An aorto-oesophageal fistula presents with massive and fatal bleeding.

The diagnosis is confirmed by:

– chest radiograph
– barium swallow.

Management

- Treatment is most successful if an oesophageal stent can be placed to occlude the fistula and prevent aspiration.
- Plastic stents are the most effective but covered expandible stents are being used increasingly and have the advantages discussed above.

Further reading

1 Pasricha PJ, Fleischer DE, Kalloo AN. Endoscopic perforations of the upper digestive tract: a review of their pathogenesis, prevention and management. *Gastroenterology* 1994; **106**:787–802.

20 Peptic ulcer perforation

Clinical presentation

Classically, the patient presents with sudden, severe epigastric pain followed by generalized abdominal pain. Rarely the pain is referred to the shoulders. On examination the patient is very ill with signs of generalized peritonitis, abdomen is rigid, silent and has severe rebound tenderness. The patient usually has a tachycardia and fever. Hypotension occurs later when bacterial peritonitis develops.

The classical presentation may be modified in certain conditions. In the elderly or very young, signs and symptoms may be less severe. In the patient who is recovering from an abdominal operation for another disease, the pain and tenderness may be put down to routine postoperative events. In patients who are on steroids, the abdominal findings may be masked. Rarely, fluid may flow down the paracolic gutters producing pain in the right or left iliac fossa mimicking acute appendicitis or diverticulitis respectively. Bleeding may be present in 10–15%.

Mortality rate can be as high as 23% related to the proportion of elderly patients and to the delay in presentation or treatment.

Diagnosis

Free air under the diaphragm on the upright film or under the lateral abdominal wall on decubitus views – seen in about 75%.

Gastrograffin swallow will demonstrate free perforation.

Differential diagnosis – all causes of acute upper abdominal pain (see Chapter 4). If hypotension is seen early with the onset of pain, consider ruptured aortic aneurysm, acute pancreatitis or mesenteric infarction.

Aetiology

Peptic ulcer disease.

Perforation is the first manifestation of ulcer disease in about 2% of patients with duodenal ulcer. After the diagnosis of duodenal ulcer, perforations occur at a rate of 0·3% annually in the first 10 years. Ninety per cent of all perforated duodenal ulcers occur in the anterior wall of the duodenal bulb; 60% of perforated gastric ulcers are located on the lesser curvature and the other 40% are distributed equally on the anterior, posterior and pre-pyloric areas.

History

Ask questions to try to establish a history of dyspepsia or previous diagnosis of peptic ulcer (60–75% of patients). Previous history of perforation is present in about 7%. Ask if they have been taking aspirin or NSAIDs. Elderly people taking NSAIDs are particularly susceptible.

Examination

In the physical examination, look for pyrexia, tachycardia, hypotension, peritonitis and site of maximal tenderness.

Investigations

- Check full blood picture, amylase, urea and electroytes, calcium, liver function tests, amylase.
- Plain erect, supine abdominal x rays should be performed to look for free air (Figure 20.1). Right decubitus abdominal x rays should be performed in those who are unable to be erect.
- Gastrograffin swallow. Extravasation of contrast is seen except in the few who may have already sealed their perforation.

Management of perforated ulcer

Nil by mouth

Nasogastric tube

Fluid replacement

Intravenous fluids with normal saline to replace loss of fluid volume. Aim to achieve a diuresis of 30 ml/h. Patients with a history

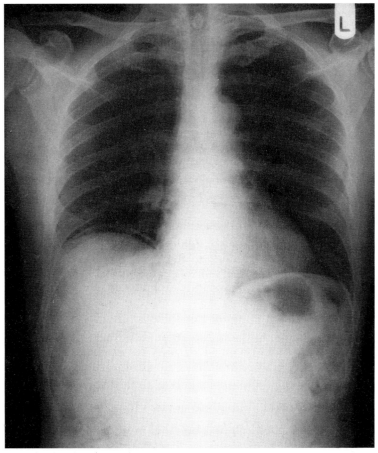

Figure 20.1 Free air under right hemidiaphragm consistent with a perforated abdominal viscus

of congestive heart failure may require central venous pressure monitoring in an intensive care setting.

Analgesia

Pethidine (Demerol) is used.

Antibiotics

Antibiotics should be given to cover Gram negative rods, Gram-positive coci and anaerobes. Broad spectrum antibiotics that provide adequate cover are: amoxycillin 1–2 G iv every 4 hs, gentamicin 1·5 mg/kg iv every 8 h and metronidazole 500 mg iv every 8 h.

Acid suppression

Administer intravenous omeprazole 40 mg iv bolus or pantoprazole 40 mg iv bolus.

Emergency surgery

- Once the decision to operate is made, there should be minimal delay to surgery (less than 2–3 h) as a long duration of perforation is the major risk factor for poor outcome.
- Most surgeons now close the perforation and perform peritoneal lavage followed by medical treatment of the ulcer, e.g. cure of *H.pylori* and proton pump inhibitor therapy.
- Definitive ulcer surgery is still performed in a few instances if proper indications exist and there are no contraindications (see Table 20.1).
- Closure of the perforation is accomplished using vascularised omentum as a patch or simple closure. Traditionally, open surgery is performed. Recently there are series reporting laparoscopic omental patch closure with good results.
- For gastric ulcers, an additional option is local excision or antrectomy because of the possibility of malignancy.
- Definitive ulcer operation (see Table 20.1) includes:
  - proximal gastric vagotomy for duodenal ulcer,
  - excision of the ulcer with vagotomy and a drainage procedure for gastric ulcer.

Postoperative care

- Nasogastric suction until the stomach begins to empty.
- Intravenous omeprazole or pantoprazole.
- *H.pylori* eradication therapy.
- Consider maintenance oral proton pump inhibition to reduce risk of recurrence.
- Postoperative antibiotics should be continued for 48 h. If intraperitoneal cultures are positive, they should be given for 7–10 days.

Table 20.1 Criteria for definitive ulcer operation for perforated ulcer.

Long history of ulcer disease, especially patients undergoing active medical treatment
Prior obstruction, haemorrhage or perforation
No concurrent medical problems
Gastric ulcers with coexistent duodenal ulcer disease
*Duration of perforation less than 24 h
*Peritoneal contamination must not be extensive
*Patient must be haemodynamically stable

*These criteria are essential

Table 20.2 Criteria for nonoperative management of perforated ulcer.

Indications
  Non surgical candidates because they are not deemed to tolerate anaesthesia
    due to multiple medical problems
  Late presentation >24–36 h after a perforation
  Stable with no signs of peritonitis
  Gastrografin swallow reveals no free leak into the peritoneal cavity

Relative contraindications
  Chronic ulcer history
  Steroids
  Gastric ulcer
  Peritonitis
  Diagnostic uncertainty
  Perforation while on adequate medical therapy

Nonoperative management

- For criteria in selecting patients for nonoperative management, please see Table 20.2.
- In selected patients, nonoperative therapies have yielded similar results to surgery.
- Nasogastric suction should be maintained.
- Intravenous omeprazole or pantoprazole (see above) should be given.
- Careful attention to fluid requirements (see above).
- Consider early institution of total parenteral nutrition.
- If fever and leukocytosis persist over several days, a CT scan of the abdomen should be obtained and any loculated fluid collection drained percutaneously. If the clinical picture does not improve, surgery will be necessary to accomplish adequate drainage.

Further reading

1 Boey J, Choi SK, Poon A, Alagartnam TT. Risk stratification in perforated duodenal ulcers: a prospective validation of predictive factors. *Ann Surg* 1987;**205**:22–6.
2 Crofts TJ, Park KGM, Steele RJC, Chung SSC, Li AKC. A randomized trial of nonoperative treatment for perforated peptic ulcer. *N Engl J Med* 1989;**320**:970–3.
3 Debas HT, Orloff SL. Surgery for peptic ulcer disease and postgastrectomy syndromes. In: Yamada T, ed. *Textbook of gastroenterology*, 2nd edn. Philadelphia: Lippincott 1995:1523–43.
4 Naesgaard JM, Edwin B, Reiertsen O, Trondsen E, Faerden AE, Rosseland AR. Laparoscopic and open operation in patients with perforated peptic ulcer. *Eur J Surg* 1999;**165**(3):209–14.

21 Gastric outlet obstruction

Clinical presentation

Patients who have obstruction from peptic ulcer disease usually have a chronic history of ulcer pain. Nausea and vomiting are present in 90% of patients with gastric outlet obstruction. Other symptoms include bloating, epigastric fullness, anorexia, unpleasant taste in the mouth, fatigue, early satiety and weight loss. In late stages the vomiting is usually after the evening meal, relieves pain and fullness, contains gastric contents or poorly digested food from a meal eaten earlier.

Physical signs include weight loss and a "succusion splash".

Diagnosis

Barium meal may show a large gastric shadow with a fluid level. A marked delay in emptying of the barium is evident with greater than 50% retention of the barium at 4 h.

Endoscopy after prolonged nasogastric drainage will show a large gastric residue with scarring of the duodenal cap. An active ulcer may be seen at the pylorus or duodenum. The pylorus is deformed and the endoscope cannot be passed easily or at all into the duodenum.

Aetiology

Please see Table 21.1. There has been a shift in incidence with more cases resulting from gastric cancer (42%) compared to peptic ulcer (37%). The incidence of obstruction in patients with peptic ulcer disease ranges from 6–22%. Obstruction is due to chronic fibrosis with acute ulceration; the former on its own rarely causes symptoms of complete obstruction.

Table 21.1 Causes of gastric outlet obstruction (common causes in italics).

Tumours
   Gastric carcinoma
   Duodenal carcinoma
   Lymphoma
   Pancreatic carcinoma
   Carcinomatosis
   Adenomatous polyp
Peptic ulcer disease
Duodenal web
Annular pancreas
Adult hypertrophic pyloric stenosis
Crohn's disease
Cholecystitis
Pancreatitis
Antral web
Eosinophilic gastroenteritis
Tuberculosis
Syphilis
Amyloidosis
Ectopic pancreas
Caustic stricture
Sarcoidosis

History

Ask questions to try to establish a history of dyspepsia or previous diagnosis of peptic ulcer. Ask if they have been taking aspirin or NSAIDs.

Examination

Look for evidence of weight loss, dehydration and a "succussion splash" (present in 25–44%). A succussion splash may be heard by the aided ear or stethoscope as the torso is moved from side to side.

Investigations

- Check full blood picture, urea and electroytes and blood gases. There may be a hypochloraemic, hypokalemic metabolic acidosis as a result of loss of hydrochloric acid from progressive vomiting. As dehydration develops, renal mechanisms are activated to conserve sodium. Both potassium and hydrogen are exchanged for sodium and the patients develop paradoxical urinary acidosis with systemic alkalosis.

- Plain abdominal x rays to look for a large gastric shadow with fluid level.
- Barium meal.
- Upper GI endoscopy after prolonged nasogastric suction.
- Barium meals and upper gastrointestinal endoscopy may provide complimentary information. Usually both investigations are performed.

Management of gastric outlet obstruction

Fluid replacement

Intravenous fluids to replace loss of fluid volume. Adequate fluid replacement must be given if there is evidence of dehydration. Normal saline is given to replace chloride loss. Potassium replacement is usually required.

Nasogastric tube

This relieves vomiting and abdominal distension. It is essential prior to carrying out endoscopy as it empties the stomach and hence reduces the risk of aspiration during the procedure.

Parenteral nutrition

Patients who have lost a significant amount of weight and are malnourished should have total parenteral nutrition.

Intravenous acid inhibition

The aim is to reduce the amount of acid volume in the stomach. If the obstruction is due to peptic ulcer, acid inhibition can accelerate ulcer healing. The most effective way to reduce acid is with intravenous omeprazole 40 mg iv once daily or pantoprazole 40 mg iv once daily.

Endoscopic therapy

Peptic ulcer disease

- Endoscopic dilatation of pyloric stenosis with balloons have been used. Sixty per cent of patients may show symptomatic relief. Ultimately 40–50% may require surgery.
- Patients with the following characteristics should be considered for surgery rather than endoscopic treatment:

111

- active, possibly penetrating channel ulcer
- long stenosis
- possibility of malignancy
- congenital abnormality
- need for repeated dilatation
- inadequate resolution of symptoms following dilatation.

Gastric cancer

- There is encouraging initial experience in the use of duodenal stents for palliation with good results particularly in patients who are high risk surgical candidates.

Surgery

Peptic ulcer disease (Figure 21.1)

- The goal of surgery is to alleviate gastric outlet obstruction and to consider treating the underlying disease by a vagotomy. Most surgeons do not now perform a vagotomy but instead treat conservatively with proton pump inhibitor therapy.

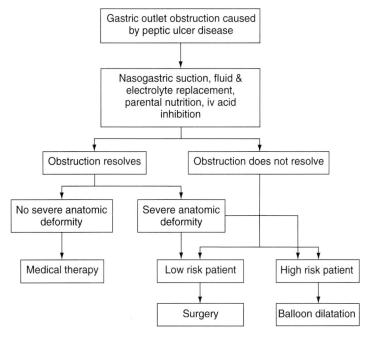

Figure 21.1 Recommmendations for treatment of obstructing peptic ulcer disease.

Gastric cancer

- Where possible a curative operation is undertaken.
- If the cancer has spread to involve the liver or vital structures to make it unresectable, then a palliative drainage procedure is undertaken.

Further reading

1 Brunner GH, Thiesemann C. The potential clinical role of intravenous omeprazole. *Digestion* 1992;**51**(Suppl 1):17–20.
2 Kozarek RA. Endotherapy for gastric outlet obstruction. *Gastrointest Endosc* 1996;**43**:173–4.
3 Pappas TN, Lapp JA. Complications of peptic ulcer disease: perforation and obstruction. In: Taylor MD, ed. *Gastrointestinal emergencies*, 2nd edn. Baltimore: Williams & Wilkins, 1997: 87–98.

22 Nonvariceal haemorrhage

PEPTIC ULCER BLEEDING

Introduction

Haemorrhage is the most common complication of peptic ulcers occurring in approximately 15% of ulcer patients. It tends to be more common in patients aged 60 and older. Approximately 10–20% of peptic ulcers bleed without any antecedent symptoms.

History, examination, investigations

Please see Chapter 3.

Management of haemorrhage from peptic ulcer

General measures

Please see Chapter 3.

Pharmacotherapy

- Proton pump inhibitors – their administration may result in better outcome such as reduced blood transfusion requirement, surgery and complications in patients with ulcers showing stigmata of recent haemorrhage, compared to placebo in two of three prospective placebo controlled randomized trials. Omeprazole 40 mg iv daily and pantoprazole 40 mg iv daily are available as intravenous preparations in some countries and may be given to those who are on nil by mouth.
- Eradication of *H. pylori* if present reduces the risk of recurrent ulcers and bleeding.

Endoscopic therapy

- Timing of endoscopy is discussed in Chapter 3.
- Endoscopic stigmata of recent haemorrhage can predict the risk of rebleeding and need for endoscopic haemostasis or surgery (see Table 22.1 and Plates 1–5).
- Endoscopic methods for haemostasis are listed in Table 22.2.
- In the best hands, initial haemostasis can be achieved in 90–100% of ulcers with active bleeding or visible vessels. About 20–40% require repeat injections for rebleeding and 5–28% require emergency surgery. Many studies have shown that compared to medical therapy alone, outcome such as need for blood transfusions, need for surgery, hospital stay, cost and perhaps mortality are reduced.
- There appears to be little difference in efficacy between the methods of haemostasis used. The choice of the method used is dependent on local expertise. The most popular methods are bipolar coagulation and injection therapy with 1:10 000 adrenaline. A combination of these two methods may have particular enhanced benefit for a subgroup with arterial bleeding.
- Patients with active arterial bleeding or visible vessel who are treated endoscopically with successful haemostasis should be considered for repeat endoscopy and retreatment if necessary after 24 h.
- If patients rebleed despite initial successful endoscopic therapy, consideration should be given for either repeat endoscopic therapy or surgery.

Table 22.1 Rebleeding rates and need for endoscopic treatment based on endoscopic stigmata of recent haemorrhage.

Endoscopic stigmata	Incidence (%)	Risk of rebleeding (%)	Endoscopic Treatment?
Active arterial bleeding	5–15	90–100	Yes
Visible vessel	25	50	Yes
Adherent clot	15	30	Yes*
Flat/red black spots	15–20	5–10	No
No stigmata	35	0–3	No

*Initial results from a prospective randomised study suggests that where endoscopic expertise is available, firmly adherent clots should be forcibly removed and the underlying ulcer treated endoscopically.

Table 22.2 Endoscopic methods for haemostasis of nonvariceal haemorrhage

Method	Delivery
Thermally active methods	Electrocoagulation Bipolar Monopolar Heater probe Laser
Injection	Adrenaline 1:10 000 Tissue glues
Mechanical methods	Endoscopic clips Band ligation
Combination methods	Inject + thermal

Surgery

- Indications for surgery include:
  - Failure to stabilise haemodynamically despite aggressive fluid resuscitation and 4 units of packed red blood cells.
  - Failure of endoscopic techniques to arrest haemorrhage.
  - Recurrent haemorrhage after initial endoscopic haemostasis in the elderly or unfit or after two attempts at endoscopic control in young fit patients.
  - Continued slow haemorrhage requiring 3 units transfusion per day.
- Surgery for haemorrhage from duodenal ulcer involves over-sewing or excision of the ulcer followed by postoperative *H. pylori* eradication.
- Surgery for haemorrhage from gastric ulcer involves a partial distal gastrectomy with Billroth I anastomosis.

Follow-up post discharge

- Proton pump inhibitors should be prescribed for 2 months or more in certain situations.
- All patients with gastric ulcer should have repeat endoscopy in 4 weeks to ensure healing.
- If *H. pylori* is present, it should be cured by one of the following regimens:
  1 week treatment with:
  - proton pump inhibitor bd + clarithromycin 500 mg bd + amoxycillin 1 g bd

- proton pump inhibitor bd + clarithromycin 500 mg bd + metronidazole 400 mg bd
- proton pump inhibitor bd + metronidazole 400 mg bd + amoxycillin 1 g bd.
- Cure of *H.pylori* should be confirmed 4 weeks after treatment with a C13 urea breath test for duodenal ulcer or repeat endoscopy for gastric ulcer.
- NSAIDs should be stopped if possible. If not, patients should receive concomitant proton pump inhibitors.

GASTRITIS AND GASTRIC EROSIONS

Clinical presentation

Endoscopically, gastritis is defined by the gross appearance of mucosal haemorrhages, erythema and erosions. An erosion is defined as an area of adherent haemorrhage or a defect in the mucosa that is less than 3–5 mm and without significant depth.

Most bleeding from NSAID induced erosive gastritis usually resolves spontaneously. In the alcoholic, portal hypertensive gastropathy can occur as a result of portal hypertension. Severe cases of portal hypertensive gastropathy can be associated with overt and chronic bleeding. Stress induced gastritis can result in significant bleeding. When this occurs, it is associated with high treatment failure rates and significant morbidity.

History, examination, investigations

Please see Chapter 3.

Management of gastritis and gastric erosions

General measures

Please see Chapter 3.

Pharmacological therapy

- Proton pump inhibitors and/or sucralfate 1 g qid are commonly administered for erosive gastritis and may have marginal efficacy in the treatment of the bleeding.
- Propranolol to reduce portal pressure is the treatment of choice in portal hypertensive gastropathy and can decrease rebleeding based on two controlled studies.

- Intravenous infusion of vasopressin (20 units over 15 min) has been reported to be effective in those with severe haemorrhage although is not well studied.

Endoscopic therapy

This is the first and safest choice of treatment in those with significant bleeding from stress gastritis. It has not been specifically studied in this context. Modalities such as bipolar coagulation, heater probe, injection of adrenaline or sclerosant can be tried. The presence of multiple bleeding sites precludes its use.

Angiography

Angiographic control of gastric mucosal bleeding reportedly has a good success rate. Intraarterial vasopressin controls haemorrhage in 80–90% of the successfully catheterized gastritis patients. However only 75% of these patients can be successfully catheterized.

Surgery

The operative mortality is extremely high and rebleeding after surgery is common. It should be reserved as a last alternative.

MALLORY–WEISS TEAR

Clinical presentation

Mallory–Weiss tears occur near the gastroesophageal junction in gastric or oesophageal mucosa. They are caused by retching. There is usually a history of vomiting foodstuffs before haematemesis although the blood can occur with the first vomitus. Many have a history of alcohol intake or have portal hypertension.

Management

- The bleeding usually resolves with conservative management.
- In those whose bleeding does not stop or they rebleed, endoscopic therapy with bipolar coagulation or injection with adrenaline can be effective.
- Other options include intraarterial vasopressin or oversewing of the bleeding mucosa.

OESOPHAGITIS AND OESOPHAGEAL ULCERS

Clinical presentation

The main cause of these is reflux disease. Rarer causes include radiation therapy, infection, e.g. herpesvirus, pill-induced damage, sclerotherapy or band ligation of varices.

Management

- Pharmacological therapy with proton pump inhibitors. Sucralfate can also be added.
- Bleeding in the majority will stop spontaneously. However persistent or recurrent bleeding should be treated with endoscopic therapy such as bipolar coagulation or injection with adrenaline.

CANCER

Clinical presentation

Bleeding from these lesions is usually self-limited.

Management

- Treatment is usually in the hands of the oncologist or surgeon.
- If persistent or recurrent bleeding occurs in a patient unsuitable for surgery, endoscopic therapy (with bipolar coagulation or argon plasma coagulation), or angiographic arterial embolisation may be used.

VASCULAR MALFORMATIONS

Angiodysplasia and hereditary haemorrhagic telangiectasiae

Clinical presentation

Most of these patients present with gastrointestinal haemorrhage (Plate 6). Typical clinical features that help identify the patient with hereditary haemorrhagic telangiectasiae includes family history,

119

telangiectasiaes on the lips, oral and nasopharyngeal membranes, tongue and hands and pulmonary arteriovenous fistulas.

Management

- Endoscopic coagulation techniques (bipolar coagulation or argon plasma coagulation or laser) can be successful although it may be associated with high rebleeding rates.
- Angiography can be used to localise small bowel lesions.
- Surgical resection may be performed if the bleeding lesion is identified clearly.
- Oestrogen-progesterone therapy has been reported to be beneficial although is poorly tolerated.

Dieulafoy's lesion

Clinical presentation

The Dieulafoy's lesion is a ruptured, thick-walled artery with little or no associated ulceration. It occurs in the fundus. It is uncommon but is seen in 1–2% of patients presenting with massive upper gastrointestinal haemorrhage.

Management

- Diagnosis is made by endoscopy performed when the patient is actively bleeding. The Dieulafoy lesion appears as a round mucosal defect with a protruding artery at the base.
- It is treated by endoscopic injection therapy with ethanolamine, electrocoagulation, or band ligation.
- Surgery is occasionally required.

AORTOENTERIC FISTULA

Clinical presentation

Most aortoenteric fistulas are secondary to prior aortic Dacron graft surgery. The fistulas almost always involve the third portion of the duodenum. The classical presentation is a "herald" bleed that occurs and stops spontaneously hours or occasionally weeks before the major haemorrhage.

Management

- A high index of suspicion is necessary to make the diagnosis.
- The endoscopist should attempt to reach the third part of the duodenum to visualise the fistula.
- If there is a high index of suspicion, a vascular surgeon should be consulted after upper gastrointestinal endoscopy has excluded other causes of bleeding.
- Abdominal CT may demonstrate the fistula.
- Surgery is required to repair the fistula.

HAEMATOBILIA

Clinical presentation

Haematobilia is haemorrhage into the biliary tract. Haemorrhage into the pancreatic duct is called haemosuccus pancreaticus. The most common cause of haematobilia is prior liver or biliary tree trauma, e.g. from a liver biopsy. Less common causes include hepatic tumours, gallstones and cholecystitis. Haemosuccus pancreaticus occurs due to peripancreatic pseudoaneurysm, pseudocyst and venous rupture, true aneurysms of peripancreatic vessels.

Management

- The diagnosis is made by endoscopy with visualisation of blood coming from the papilla.
- Angiography is indicated to define the bleeding site and embolisation of the vessel may stop the haemorrhage.
- If angiography is not successful, surgery may be required.

Further reading

1 Athanasoulis CA, Baum S, Waltman AC, *et al.* Control of acute mucosal hemorrhage. Intraarterial infusion of posterior pituitary extract. *N Engl J Med* 1974;**290**:597.
2 Chung SCS, Leung JWC, Steele RJC, Crofts TI, Li AKC. Endoscopic injection of adrenaline for actively bleeding ulcers: a randomized trial. *Br Med J* 1988;**296**:1631–3.
3 Elta GH. Approach to the patient with gross gastrointestinal bleeding. In: Yamada T, ed. *Textbook of gastroenterology*, 2nd edn. Philadelphia: Lippincott, 1995:671–98.
4 Jaspersen D, Koerner T, Schorr W, Brennenstuhl M, Raschka C, Hammar C-H. *Helicobacter pylori*: eradication reduces the rate of rebleeding in ulce hemorrhage. *Gastrointest Endosc* 1995;**41**:5–7.
5 Jensen DM, Machicado GA, Kovacs TOG, *et al.* Controlled randomized study of heater probe and BICAP for hemostasis of severe ulcer bleeding [abstract]. *Gastroenterology* 1988;**94**:A208.
6 Khuroo MS, Yattoo GN, Javid G *et al.* A comparison of omeprazole and placebo for bleeding peptic ulcer. *N Engl J Med* 1997;**336**(15):1054–8

7 Perez-Ayuso RM, Pigue JM, Bosch J, *et al.* Propranolol in prevention of recurrent bleeding from severe portal hypertensive gastropathy on cirrhosis. *Lancet* 1991;**337**:1431.
8 Semb BKH, Sejonsby H, Solhaug JH. Intravenous infusion of vasopressin in the treatment of bleeding from severe hemorrhagic gastritis. *Acta Chir Scand* 1983;**149**:579.

23 Acute pancreatitis

Clinical presentation

Epigastric pain usually radiating to the back occurs in 95% of patients. Nausea and vomiting occur in 85%. Low grade fevers occur in 60%. Tachycardia and hypotension occur in 40%. Abdominal tenderness and guarding with decreased or absent bowel sounds are common. Mild jaundice is not unusual.

Diagnosis

Serum amylase level of > 1000 IU/l is diagnostic.

Raised amylase < 1000 IU/l may also occur in perforated peptic ulcer, acute cholecystitis leaking aortic aneurysm, renal failure, ischaemic bowel, ruptured ectopic pregnancy.

Serum lipase is as sensitive and more specific than amylase. It remains elevated longer than the amylase level and may help to diagnose acute pancreatitis after an acute attack has passed.

Aetiology

Gallstones or microlithiasis
Alcohol } both account for 80%

Other causes

Structural – pancreas divisum, trauma.
Drugs   – azathioprine, 6-mercaptopurine, asparaginase, pentamidine, 2′,2′-dideoxyinosine.
Infection – viral (mumps, coxsackie), bacteria, parasites (ascaris).
Vascular   – atherosclerosis, vasculitis.
Others   – hyperlipidaemia, coronary bypass, cystic fibrosis,

fibrocalculous, hypercalcaemia, iatrogenic, inflammatory bowel disease, neoplasia, peptic ulcer, hereditary, idiopathic.

Prediction of severity of pancreatitis

It is important to predict the severity in acute pancreatitis because:

- It allows the clinician to predict the patient's course and direct appropriate placement of the patient, e.g. ICU in severe pancreatitis.
- Allows consideration of intervention, e.g. ERCP.

The definition of severe pancreatitis is based on the presence of organ failure (hypoxia, renal compromise, hypotension, gastrointestinal bleeding) and/or local complications (e.g. necrosis) (see Table 23.1).

Mortality is close to zero when there are 0–1 indicators of organ failure but >19% when there are 2 or more indicators of organ failure.

Several scoring systems have been devised to predict severity (see Tables 23.1–23.4). The disadvantage of Ranson's criteria is that they require 11 values be monitored over 48 hours of measurement. The simplified Glasgow criteria has the advantage that they can be calculated any time within the first 48 h and measure only eight parameters. The advantage of the APACHE is that it can be calculated instantaneously from routine measurements and can be regularly updated to follow a patient's progress. A major disadvantage is that it is complex and requires computer analysis to establish a prognostic score.

History

Ask questions to try to establish the aetiology of the pancreatitis, e.g. a history of biliary colic which may suggest gallstones, heavy alcohol intake which may suggest alcoholic pancreatitis, drug history.

Table 23.1 Indicators of organ failure.

Hypotension – systolic BP < 90 mm Hg
Hypoxia – $PaO_2 \leq 8kPa$ (60 mm Hg)
Renal failure – creatinine > 200 μmol/l (2 mg/dl)
GI bleeding – > 500 ml/24 h

Table 23.2 Ranson's prognostic scoring criteria.

At admission
Age > 55 years
WBC >16 000 /mm3
Glucose >200 mg/dl (10 mmol/l)
LDH >350 IU/l
AST >250 U/l

During initial 48 h
Haematocrit decrease of > 10
Urea increase of >5 mg/dl
Calcium < 8 mg/dl (2 mmol/l)
PaO_2 < 60 mm Hg (8 kPa)
Base deficit >4 mEq/l
Fluid sequestration >6l

Signs	Morbidity (%)	Mortality (%)
<2	<5	<1
3–5	30	5
>6	90	20

Table 23.3 Simplified Glasgow prognostic scoring criteria.

During initial 48 h

Age > 55 years
WBC >15 000 mm^3
LDH >600 IU/l
Glucose > 180 mg/dl (10 mmol/l)
Albumin < 32 g/l
Calcium < 8 mg/dl (2.0 mmol/l)
PaO_2 < 60 mm Hg (8 kPa)
Urea >45 mg/dl (16 mmol/l)

> 3 signs indicates severe attack.

Examination

- Abdominal findings may include tenderness in the epigastrium with rebound and guarding, absent bowel sounds.
- Assess the presence of dyspnoea which may indicate hypoxia, temperature, jaundice, blood pressure, dark discolouration in the back (Grey–Turner's sign) or periumbilical region (Cullen's sign).

Table 23.4 APACHE-II severity of disease classification system. Eight or more points indicates severe pancreatitis.

Physiologic variable	High abnormal range				0	Low abnormal range			
	+4	+3	+2	+1		+1	+2	+3	+4
1. Temperature – rectal (°C)	≥41°	39°–40.9°		38.5°–38.9°	36°–38.4°	34°–35.9°	32°–33.9°	30°–31.9°	≤29.9°
2. Mean arterial pressure (mm Hg)	≥160	130–159	110–129		70–109		50–69		≤49
3. Heart rate (ventricular response)	≥180	140–179	110–139		70–109		55–69	40–54	≤39
4. Respiratory rate (nonventilated or ventilated)	≥50	35–49		25–34	12–24	10–11	6–9		≤5
5. Oxygenation: A-aDO$_2$ or PaO$_2$ (mm Hg)									
a. FIO$_2$ ≥ 0.5: record A-aDO$_2$	≥500	350–499	200–349		<200				
b. FIO$_2$ < 0.5: record only PaO$_2$				PO$_2$ 61–70	PO$_2$ >70			PO$_2$ 55–60	PO$_2$ <55
6. Arterial ph	≥7.7	7.6–7.69		7.5–7.59	7.33–7.49		7.25–7.32	7.15–7.24	<7.15
7. Serum sodium (mmol/L)	≥180	160–179	155–159	150–154	130–149		120–129	111–119	<110
8. Serum potassium (mmol/L)	≥7	6–6.9		5.5–5.9	3.5–5.4	3–3.4	2.5–2.9		<2.5
9. Serum creatinine (mg/100 mL) (Double point score for acute renal failure)	≥3.5	2–3.4	1.5–1.9		0.6–1.4		<0.6		
10. Hematocrit (%)	≥60		50–59.9	46–49.9	30–45.9		20–29.9		<20
11. White blood count (total/mm³) (in 1000 sec)	≥40		20–39.9	15–19.9	3–14.9		1–2.9		<1
12. Glasgow coma score (GCS): Score = 15 minus actual GCS									
13. Total Acute physiology score (APS) Sum of the 12 individual variable points									
14. Serum HCO$_2$ (venous: mmol/L) (Not preferred, use if no ABGs)	≥52	41–51.9		32–40.9	22–31.9		18–21.9	15–17.9	<15

Percentage Points

Assign points to age as follows:

Age (years)	Points
≤44	0
45–54	2
55–64	3
65–74	5
≥75	6

Chronic health points

If the patient has a history of severe organ system insufficiency or immunocompromised, assign points as follows:

For nonoperative or emergency postoperative patients: 5 points

or

For elective postoperative patients: 2 points

Definitions: Organ insufficiency or immunocompromised state must have been evident prior to this hospital admission and conforms to the following criteria:

Liver: Biopsy-proven cirrhosis and documented portal hypertension, episodes of past upper GI bleeding attributed to portal hypertension; or prior episodes of hepatic failure/encephalopathy/coma.

Cardiovascular: NY Heart Association Class IV.

Respiratory: Chronic restrictive, obstructive, or vascular disease resulting in severe exercise restriction (e.g. unable to climb stairs or perform household duties); or documented chronic hypoxia, hypercapnia, secondary polycythemia, severe pulmonary hypertension (>40 mm Hg), or respirator dependency.

Renal: Recurring chronic dialysis.

Immunocompromised: The patient has received therapy that suppresses resistance to infection (e.g. immunosuppression, chemotherapy, radiation, long term or recent high-dose steroids) or has a disease that is sufficiently advanced to suppress resistance to infection (e.g. leukemia, lymphoma, AIDS).

APACHE-II score
Sum of A + B + C

A APS points _____

B Age points _____

C Chronic health points _____

Total Apache-II score _____

Severe pancreatitis if score ≥8

Investigations

- Check full blood picture, amylase, lipase, urea and electroytes, calcium, liver function tests, arterial blood gases, LDH, lipid profile.
- Ultrasound scan should be performed on the next available list to evaluate the biliary tract and detect gallstones, bile duct dilatation, cholecystitis, sludge in gallbladder
- CT scan – dynamic contrast enhanced CT is a good prognostic indicator (Table 23.5). The routine use of CT is not justified except in patients with severe pancreatitis.

Management of acute pancreatitis

Severity of pancreatitis

Predict severity of pancreatitis using the criteria described above. If pancreatitis is severe, consider managing the patient in an intensive care setting (see Figure 23.1).

Fluid replacement

Intravenous fluids to prevent hypovolaemia. The haemodynamic upset is similar to that of septic shock with decreased peripheral resistance and elevation in cardiac index.

Table 23.5 Computed tomography severity index.

Grade of acute pancreatitis	Points
A: Normal pancreas	0
B: Pancreatic enlargement	1
C: Inflammation confined to pancrease and peripancreatic fat	2
D: One peripancreatic fluid collection	3
E: Two or more fluid collections	4
Degree of necrosis	
No necrosis	0
Necrosis of one third of pancreas	2
Necrosis of one half of pancreas	4
Necrosis of more than one half	6

Computed tomography severity index = grade points + degree of necrosis

Points	Morbidity (%)	Mortality (%)
<2	4	0
7–10	92	17

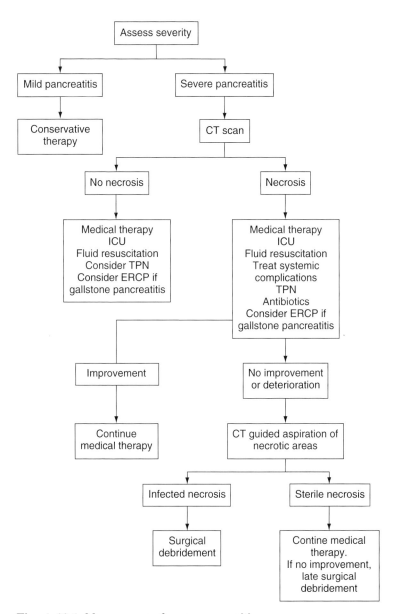

Figure 23.1 Management of acute pancreatitis.

Urine volume should be monitored hourly after urinary catheterisation.

Analgesia

Pethidine (Demerol) is used.

Nutritional support

- Initially the patient should have nil by mouth.
- In mild pancreatitis, when the patient starts to feel hungry, oral feeding can commence.
- In severe pancreatitis, if it is likely that the patient will not be fed orally for a significant period, parenteral feeding should be started.
- An alternative means of feeding the patient is to insert a naso-jejunal feeding tube distal to the pancreas.

Nasogastric suction

This should be used if the patient has severe pancreatitis and an ileus.

Respiratory support

If the patient is hypoxic, they should receive oxygen. In severe hypoxia and respiratory distress, assisted ventilator therapy may be indicated.

Antibiotics

- Should only be used in the presence of necrotising pancreatitis diagnosed by dynamic CT, cholangitis or predicted severe pancreatitis.
- A cephalosporin, e.g. cefuroxime 1·5 g tid iv is used in either situation.
- An alternative antibiotic, imipenem 500 mg tid iv can be used in necrotising pancreatitis but is more expensive.
- Randomised clinical trials have shown improved outcome with reduction in sepsis, morbidity and mortality if these are used in necrotising pancreatitis.

ERCP

- Urgent ERCP and endoscopic sphincterotomy within 72 h is indicated in the following situations:
  - Coexistent cholangitis (jaundice, pyrexia, gallstones).
  - Predicted severe gallstone pancreatitis.

- Initial mild gallstone pancreatitis that is not resolving or deteriorating.
- Randomised clinical trials have shown that in these situations, morbidity and perhaps mortality can be reduced.
- Non urgent ERCP should be considered in the following situations:
  - Mild gallstone pancreatitis – this should be performed after the pancreatitis has settled.
  - Idiopathic pancreatitis – performed if there is strong suspicion of a bile duct stone (e.g. status post cholecystectomy, dilated bile ducts on scan, abnormal liver function tests). If suspicion of bile duct stone or carcinoma is low, it is debatable whether it should be performed after a first attack or wait until a recurrent attack.

Prevention of recurrent gallstone pancreatitis: cholecystectomy or sphincterotomy

- In gallstone pancreatitis, cholecystectomy is recommended in most cases to prevent further attacks of pancreatitis (from 30–50% to 0–5%). For cases of mild pancreatitis, the cholecystectomy should be performed at the index admission once the clinical and biochemical abnormalities have normalised. Patients with severe pancreatitis may benefit from a delay in cholecystectomy.
- Endoscopic sphincterotomy by itself without cholecystectomy is indicated in patients who are unfit for surgery.

Management of local complications

Pancreatic necrosis

- This occurs in about 20% of cases of pancreatitis. This is best confirmed by dynamic CT. See Table 23.4.
- The most serious outcome of necrosis is infection.
- Infection can be prevented by administration of cephalosporins or imipenem (see above, Antibiotics).
- Infected necrosis is heralded by a sudden increase in abdominal tenderness, high fever, marked leukocystosis and bacteremia with signs of sepsis.
- Detection of infection is made by CT guided needle aspiration (safe and reliable). Samples should be sent for Gram's stain and culture. Gram negative and anaerobic oranisms are most common.

- Treatment of infected necrosis is immediate surgery with debridement which reduces mortality from 100% to 15%.
- Treatment of sterile necrosis is more controversial. Mortality is 10%. If it is associated with prolonged or increasing systemic complications, the options are continuation of aggressive medical therapy in intensive care or early surgical debridement. Most would refrain from surgery in the absence of infection for at least 3–4 weeks until systemic toxicity has resolved.

Pseudocyst

- Acute pancreatic fluid collections are found in 30–50% of patients with severe pancreatitis (Figure 23.2); more than half will regress spontaneously.
- A fluid collection should be defined as a pseudocyst only if it persists for more than 4 weeks. It occurs in 10% of patients.
- Uncomplicated pseudocysts > 6 cm persisting > 6 weeks should be treated.
- Asymptomatic pseudocysts < 6 cm should be followed; most will resolve spontaneously.
- Treatment options for pseudocysts include:
  - Endoscopic treatment – insertion of pancreatic stent if it communicates with a pseudocyst (ERCP) or cystgastrostomy or cystduodenostomy.
  - Percutaneous drainage.
  - Surgery – cystgastrostomy, Roux-en-Y cystojejunostomy, cystoduodenostomy.
- There are no randomised controlled trials comparing these treatments, all of which have been shown to be effective in separate series. The optimal therapy has to take into account local expertise, site of the pseudocyst, whether it communicates with the pancreatic duct and presence of complications such as infection.

Fistulas

- This can result in ascites, pleural effusions or communicate with the skin (cutaneous), bowel, and other nearby structures.
- Fluid from a pancreatic fistula has high amylase and protein content. It arises from a break in the pancreatic duct or ruptured pseudocyst.
- Drainage of fluid collections by thoracentesis or paracentesis helps to heal the fistula.
- Treatment options include:

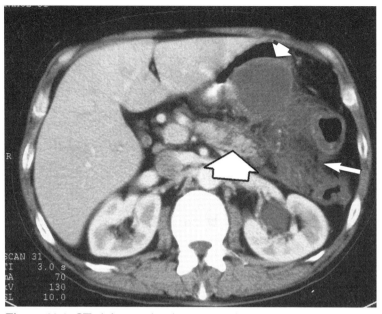

Figure 23.2 CT abdomen showing pancreatic pseudocyst (small arrow) secondary to acute pancreatitis. In the pancreas (large arrow), there is a necrotic area in the middle of the body. The margins of the pancreas are not clearly defined indicating inflammation. There are inflammatory changes in the peri pancreatic fat (thin arrow) around the region of the tail of the pancreas.

- ERCP – pancreatic stent can be inserted to reduce gradient across sphincter to allow healing of break or inserted across the break to occlude it.
- Infusion of somatostatin or octreotide (300–600 mcg daily).
- Pancreatic resection.

Management of Systemic Complications
Pulmonary

Pleural effusions are drained only if the size results in respiratory compromise as most resolve spontaneously.

Pancreatic-pleural fistulas resulting in effusions usually do not form acutely (see Fistulas above).

In patients with severe acute respiratory distress syndrome (ARDS), respiratory support with positive end expiratory pressure is required.

Gastrointestinal haemorrhage

Serious haemorrhage may arise from an abscess or pseudocyst that erodes into vascular structures. This may be treated with angiography and embolization.

Colon obstruction

Obstruction may result secondary to spasm and oedema. This is treated as for colonic obstruction (see Chapter 34).

Spleen and splenic vein

Splenic vein thrombosis may lead to splenomegaly, oesophageal, gastric varices. The preferred treatment is splenectomy.

Extension of a pseudocyst into the spleen may lead to splenic rupture. Prophylactic splenectomy has been advocated.

Further reading

1　Balthazar EJ, Robinson DL, Megibow AJ, Ranson JHC. Acute pancreatitis: value of CT in establishing prognosis. *Radiology* 1990;**174**:331–6.

2　Banks PA. A new classification system for acute pancreatitis. *Am J Gastroenterol* 1994;**89**:151–2.

3　Bradley EL, Allen K. A prospective longitudinal study of observation versus surgical intervention in the management of necrotizing pancreatitis. *Am J Surg* 1991;**161**:19.

4　Fan S-T, Lai ECS, Mok FPT, *et al.* Early treatment of acute biliary pancreatitis by endoscopic papillotomy. *N Engl J Med* 1993;**328**:228–32.

5　Gerzof SG, Banks PA, Robbins AH, *et al.* Early diagnosis of pancreatic infection by computed tomography-guided aspiration. *Gastroenterology* 1987;**93**:1315–20.

6　Neoptolemos JP, Carr-Locke DL, London NJ, *et al.* Controlled trial of urgent endoscopic retrograde cholangiopancreatography and endoscopic sphincterotomy versus conservative treatment for acute pancreatitis due to gallstones. *Lancet* 1988;**2**:979–83.

7　Pederzoli P, Bassi C, Vesentini S, Campedelli A. A randomized multicenter clinical trial of antibiotic prophylaxis of septic complications in acute necrotizing pancreatitis with imipenem. *Surg Gynecol Obstet* 1993;**176**:480.

8　Sainio V, Kemppainen E, Puolakkainen P, *et al.* Early antibiotic treatment in acute necrotising pancreatitis. *Lancet* 1995;**346**(8976):663–7

9　Wilson C, Heath DI, Imrie CW. Prediction of outcome in acute pancreatitis: a comparative study of APACHE-II, clinical asssessment and multiple factor scoring systems. *Br J Surg* 1990;**77**:1260–4.

10　United Kingdom guidelines for the management of acute pancreatitis. British Society of Gastroenterology. *Gut* 1998; 42 suppl. 2: S1–13.

24 Acute cholecystitis

Clinical presentation

Upper abdominal pain (epigastrium or right upper quadrant) is the most common presenting symptom. In the elderly, patients receiving steroids or immunocompromised; symptoms can be mild or nonspecific. Approximately two thirds of patients will have had previous episodes of biliary colic. In contrast to biliary colic, pain from acute cholecystitis is persistent and lasts more than 4–6 h (about 1–3 h in biliary colic). They may present with chest pain suggestive of myocardial ischaemia. Anorexia, nausea and vomiting are frequently present.

On physical examination, the temperature is mildly elevated. There is right upper quadrant tenderness. A palpable gallbladder is found in about a third of patients. Often a positive Murphy's sign (arrest of inspiration by the patient when the inflamed gallbladder comes in contact with the hand of the examiner pressing the right upper quadrant) is present.

Approximately 25% of patients will develop severe cholecystitis (persistent or progressive symptoms) or a complication. Mortality overall is 5%; in the young is less than 1% and elderly > 10%.

Diagnosis

Abdominal ultrasound scan – major criteria for diagnosis of acute cholecystitis include the presence of gallstones and a nonvisuallised gallbladder. Minor criteria are gallbladder wall thickening (> 4 mm), tenderness of the gallbladder induced by the ultrasound probe (sonographic Murphy's sign), gallbladder enlargement (> 5 cm), a round gallbladder shape and evidence of pericholecystic fluid. Sensitivity of major criteria for acute cholecystitis is 80–85%

and specificity between 94–98% with addition of minor criteria increasing the sensitivity.

Nuclear HIDA (hepato-imino diacetic acid) scan – performed if ultrasound study is equivocal or negative in a patient with a high index of clinical suspicion. If the gallbladder is not visualised after delayed views or injection of morphine, even with normal excretion into the intestine, the test is considered positive for acute cholecystitis. False positive scans can occur in the setting of biliary pancreatitis, liver disease, prolonged fasting and total parenteral nutrition.

See Tables 24.1 and 24.2 for differential diagnoses.

Aetiology

Ninety per cent of acute cholecystitis are associated with gallstones and the remaining cases are acalculous.

Causes of acalculous cholecystitis include: serious illness or trauma requiring bedrest, prolonged fasting, parenteral nutrition, mechanical ventilation, major surgery, multiple blood transfusions, large dosages of antibiotics, narcotics. It most commonly occurs in patients in intensive care units. It can present *de novo* in: elderly males with atherosclerosis, or those with AIDS, vasculitis.

History

In the history, ask questions to try to establish a history of biliary colic or previous diagnosis of gallstones.

Table 24.1 Differential diagnosis of acute cholecystitis.

Acute appendicitis
Acute pancreatitis
Peptic ulcer
Hepatitis
Pneumonia
Pulmonary embolism
Renal stones
Gonococcal perihepatitis
Hepatic abscess
Hepatic tumours
Coronary artery disease

Table 24.2 Differential diagnosis of air in the biliary system.

Inflammatory causes
   Cholecystitis with perforation
   Pancreatitis
   Perforated ulcer
   Recently passed common duct stone
   Crohn's disease
   Pleural effusions

Surgical
   Sphincterotomy
   Biliary intestinal anastomosis

Malignancy
   Pancreatic, ampullary, or duodenal cancer
   Metastatic disease

Infections
   Strongyloidiasis
   Clonorchis sinensis
   Ascaris lumbricoides

Emphysematous cholecystitis

Examination

In the physical examination, look for evidence of right upper quadrant tenderness, Murphy's sign.

Investigations

- Blood tests.
  - Full blood picture – Leukocytosis is present in 75% of cases
  - Liver function tests – mild nonspecific elevations in ALT (alanine aminotransferase) and AST (aspartate aminotransferase) occur in 40%. ALP (alkaline phosphatase) is elevated in the absence of a common bile duct stone in 15% of cases. When the level of the ALP is three to four times greater than normal, there is an increased probability of an associated common bile duct stone. Jaundice can be found in approximately 25% of patients in the absence of common bile duct stones.
  - Amylase – moderate hyperamylasaemia is present in a minority without pancreatitis.
  - Blood cultures.
- Abdominal x ray – gallstones will be detected in 15–20% of cases. Air in the biliary tree may be detected (see Table 24.1).

137

Other causes of abdominal pain such as obstruction or perforation can be ruled out.

- Abdominal ultrasound (see above).
- Nuclear (HIDA) scan or CT abdomen is performed if the diagnosis is still unclear.

Management of acute cholecystitis

Intravenous fluids

Nil by mouth

Nasogastric suction

Consider this if the patient is vomiting or has abdominal distension.

Antibiotics

See Table 24.3 for likely organisms.

Mild cases – intravenous cefotaxime 1 g tid or co-amoxiclav 1 g tid, for 7 days.

Severe cases – broad spectrum cover with intravenous ampicillin 500 mg tid + gentamicin (dose titrated according to body weight) + metronidazole 500 mg tid or ciprofloxacin 400 mg iv bd or 500 mg oral bd.

Surgery

- Cholecystectomy is the definitive therapy for acute cholecystitis.
- Timing of surgery – Prospective randomised trials have shown that early cholecystectomy (within 24–48 h) compared to delayed cholecystectomy (6–8 weeks later) is associated with a reduction in total duration of illness, shorter hospital stay, same incidence of operative complications, lower death rate. Overall cost is lower. Early cholecystectomy also decreases

Table 24.3 Commonly cultured organisms in acute cholecystitis.

E. Coli
Klebsiella
Enterococcus
Enterobacter
Pseudomonas
Clostridia
Bacteroides

morbidity and mortality in those aged > 70 years or those with diabetes. The recommendation is that cholecystectomy should be performed during the first 24–48 h of hospitalisation except in critically ill patients or patients with contraindications to early surgery. Approximately 10% will become worse requiring emergency surgery.

- Open or laparoscopic? – Laparoscopic cholecystectomy in the setting of acute cholecystitis is feasible in 50–75%. Contraindications include:
  - generalized peritonitis
  - severe cholangitis
  - severe coagulopathy
  - cancer of the gallbladder
  - end-stage cirrhosis of the liver
  - cholecystenteric fistulas
  - third trimester of pregnancy.
- Conversion rate to an open cholecystectomy is approximately 5%. Indications include:
  - scarring or adhesions
  - unclear anatomy
  - excessive bleeding
  - equivocal cholangiogram.

Cholecystostomy

- In high risk, critically ill patients with acute cholecystitis (calculous and acalculous), this is a safe and effective alternative to cholecystectomy. This can be performed percutaneously under ultrasound guidance.
- It can be followed by an elective cholecystectomy after resolution of the systemic illness in patients with associated gallstones or definitive therapy in those with acalculous cholecystitis.
- Acalculous cholecystitis usually occurs in critically ill, shocked, traumatised, or postoperative patients.

Endoscopic treatment

Endoscopic treatment may benefit a patient with acute cholecystitis with associated severe co-morbidity and an uncorrectable coagulopathy. The cystic duct can be cannulated and a stent or a nasobiliary tube can be placed into the gallbladder.

Management of local complications
Gallbladder perforation

- Approximately 10% of patients with acute cholecystitis will develop a gallbladder perforation. Sixty per cent occur in those over the age of 60. Those at risk are elderly patients with ischaemic heart disease, and also those with diabetes mellitus, acalculous cholecystitis, immunocompromised patients. Mortality is 15–20%.
- Diagnosis is made by having a high index of suspicion in high risk patients as above especially if they deteriorate following their initial presentation. Ultrasound scan and CT can be helpful.
- Medical therapy as for acute cholecystitis is instituted.
- Surgical treatment depends on the type of perforation:
  - Type I (30%) – free perforation followed by free spillage of bile into the peritoneal cavity. Immediate cholecystectomy is the preferred option. Cholecystotomy may only be possible in the critically ill patient or if there is severe inflammation surrounding the gallbladder.
  - Type II (50%) – localised perforation in which the bile spillage is contained by another viscus, omentum or by adhesions resulting in an abscess. Cholecystectomy is the preferred option. If the patient is extremely ill, a cholecystostomy and catheter drainage of the abscess can be performed.
  - Type III (20%) – chronic perforation that evolves into a cholecystenteric fistula. Treatment consists of cholecystectomy and resection of the fistula. In 8–20%, gallstone ileus can occur and the treatment is as below.

Gallstone ileus

- This is a mechanical intestinal obstruction caused by one or more gallstones. Elderly patients are at risk. The clinical manifestation of gallstone ileus is recurrent episodes of incomplete bowel obstruction as the stone lodges then moves distally to obstruct another area of the small bowel ("tumbling obstruction"). Mortality is 10–15%.
- Diagnosis is established by abdominal x ray.
  There are 4 signs:
  1 Air in the biliary tree.
  2 Partial or complete small bowel obstruction.
  3 Documentation of a calcified gallstone in the small bowel.
  4 Change in the position of a previously documented gallstone.
- Treatment consists of a two stage procedure. The first stage

relieves the immediate obstruction. The second stage removes the gallbladder and resects the fistula.

Emphysematous cholecystitis

- This is a severe, uncommon form of cholecystitis caused by gas-forming bacteria. Patients are typically older with diabetes being an additional risk. Incidence of gallstones is lower than for acute cholecystitis; in the former 72% are found to have gallstones. Clostridium, E. coli and anaerobic streptococcus are the most common organisms.
- The clinical picture can rapidly worsen. There is a high incidence of gangrene and perforation. Mortality is 15%.
- Diagnosis is established by abdominal x ray. It may reveal air in the gallbladder lumen, gallbladder wall or pericholecystic area. These findings are absent during the first 24–48 h. Abdominal ultrasound may reveal gas bubbles in the area of the gallbladder.
- Treatment consists of antibiotics that provide aerobic and anerobic coverage, intravenous fluids, followed by immediate surgery.

Empyema

- The gallbladder contains pus. The patient has a high fever, chills, increasing pain and is toxic. The white cell count is usually well above the range seen in uncomplicated acute cholecystitis ($>15\,000/mm^3$).
- Urgent surgery is indicated.

Mirizzi's syndrome

- Type I – This consists of obstruction of the common hepatic or common bile duct by a stone impacted in the cystic duct with surrounding inflammation.
- Type II – The stone can also erode into the lumen of the bile duct with the creation of a fistula.
- Ultrasound scan and ERCP can confirm the diagnosis.
- Type I is usually managed with a cholecystectomy, while type II is treated by a cholecysto-choledocho-duodenostomy.

Further reading

1 Jarvinen HJ, Hastbacka J. Early cholecystectomy for acute cholecystitis: a prospective randomized study. *Ann Surg* 1980;**191**:501–5.
2 National Institute of Health consensus development conference statement on gallstones and laparoscopic cholecystectomy. *Am J Surg* 1993;**165**:390–6.
3 Patti MG, Pellegrini CA, Taylor MB. Acute cholecystitis. In: Taylor MB, ed. *Gastrointestinal emergencies*, 2nd edn. Baltimore: Williams & Wilkins, 1997:257–73.

25 Biliary colic

Clinical presentation

Biliary colic is the main complaint in 70–80% of symptomatic patients. The pain is intermittent and severe, located in the epigastrium or right upper quadrant, less frequently in left upper quadrant, the praecordium and lower abdomen. Typically the pain has a sudden onset, rises in intensity to a plateau lasting up to 3 h. The pain may radiate to the interscapular region or right shoulder tip. Vomiting and sweating are usually associated. The patient is usually restless and unable to find a comfortable position.

History

The history as above should suggest the diagnosis of biliary colic. Consider the differential diagnosis:

- Peptic ulcers.
- Renal colic.
- Colonic pain, e.g. irritable bowel syndrome, carcinomas.
- Angina.
- Dissecting aortic aneurysm.
- Spinal neuralgia.
- Pleuritis.
- Pericarditis.
- Metabolic-C1 – esterase inhibitor deficiciency, acute intermittent porphyria.

Investigations

- Full blood picture.
- Liver function tests.
- Amylase.

- Plain abdominal *x* rays are rarely useful as only about 15% of gallstones are radio-opague.
- Ultrasound scan of abdomen – high sensitivity and specificity for gallstones.
- Upper gastrointestinal endoscopy if a peptic ulcer needs to be ruled out.

Management of biliary colic

Cholecystectomy

This is the only definitive treatment. Cholecystectomy will relieve true biliary colic. Age is not a contraindication to surgery but increased risks are encountered in patients with cardiovascular disease and liver cirrhosis.

Further reading

1 Jarvinen HJ, Hastbacka J. Early cholecystectomy for acute cholecystitis: a prospective randomized study. *Ann Surg* 1980;**191**:501–5.
2 National Institute of Health consensus development conference statement on gallstones and laparoscopic cholecystectomy. *Am J Surg* 1993;**165**:390–6.
3 Patti MG, Pellegrini CA, Taylor MB. Acute cholecystitis. In: Taylor MB, ed. *Gastrointestinal emergencies*, 2nd edn. Baltimore: Williams & Wilkins, 1997:257–73.

143

26 Cholangitis

Clinical presentation

Charcot's triad of fever/chills, pain and jaundice occurs in about 50–75% of patients with acute cholangitis. In less than 10% of patients, the addition of hypotension and mental confusion to Charcot's triad constitues Reynold's pentad. These classical features are not uniformly present and a high index of suspicion must be maintained especially in subtler situations where the bilirubin level may be only slightly elevated and fever is minimal. Pain may be mild and jaundice absent in up to 20% of patients

Physical examination reveals variable findings. Jaundice and mild tenderness are seen in many patients. Severe abdominal findings such as marked tenderness or diffuse signs are unusual and other possible diagnoses should be considered.

Diagnosis

Blood cultures may be positive in 20–60% (see Table 26.1 for list of possible organisms).

Bilirubin and liver enzymes are elevated in >80%. Liver enzymes are usually elevated in a mixed pattern (both alkaline phosphatase and transaminases).

Ultrasound scan will show biliary dilatation in many patients. It may also show the cause of obstruction such as a stone.

ERCP provides information about the cause of the obstruction and can treat the cause.

PTC is indicated instead of ERCP if ERCP is impossible or difficult such as a Roux-en-Y loop.

See Table 26.2 for differential diagnosis. Acute cholecystitis is common and often confused with cholangitis. Tenderness is more

Table 26.1 Bacteriology of acute cholangitis.

Common
  E. coli
  Klebsiella
  Enterococcus
  Bacteroides

Other organisms isolated
  Enterobacter
  Pseudomonas
  Citrobacter
  Proteus
  Serratia
  Streptococcal
  Clostridium
  Candida

AIDS cholangitis
  Cryptosporidium
  Cytomegalovirus
  Microsporidia
  Enterocytozoon bieneusi

Parasites
  Ascaris lumbricoides
  Fasciola hepatica
  Clonorchis sinensis
  Echinococcus granulosus
  Echinococcus multilocularis

Table 26.2 Differential diagnosis of cholangitis.

Acute cholecystitis
Perforated gallbladder
Torsion of the gallbladder
Mirizzi's syndrome
Acute pancreatitis
Drug-related pancreatitis
Drug-related cholangitis
Acute infective hepatitis
Metastatic disease
Hepatic abscess unrelated to cholangitis
Right lower lobe pneumonia

a feature of acute cholecystitis and a phlegmon may be palpable. Jaundice is more common in acute cholangitis. Although jaundice can occur with acute cholecystitis, it suggests a complication such as obstruction of the bile duct from Mirizzi's syndrome (see Chapter 24). A high white cell count is more often seen in cholangitis. Mild elevation of bilirubin and liver enzymes are seen in about

25% of patients with cholecystitis but more than 80% of patients with cholangitis will have higher levels of bilirubin and liver enzymes. An ultrasound scan showing a thick walled gallbladder with surrounding oedema and absence of biliary dilatation will favour the diagnosis of cholecystitis. An isotope HIDA scan would suggest cholecystitis if the gallbladder is not visualised.

Aetiology

See Table 26.3.

History

In the history, ask questions to try to establish a history of biliary colic or previous diagnosis of gallstones.

Examination

In the physical examination, look for evidence of pyrexia, right upper quadrant tenderness. Severe abdominal findings suggest another diagnosis.

Investigations

• Blood tests
  – Full blood picture – leukocytosis is present in 70% of cases. A high white cell count > 13 000/mm^3 suggests suppurative

Table 26.3 Causes of cholangitis.

Bile duct stones
Malignant bile duct stricture
Benign bile duct stricture
Papillary stenosis
Juxtapapillary diverticulum
Biliary instrumentation
Choledochoduodenostomy
Choledochojejunostomy
Congenital abnormalitis
   (choledochocoele, Caroli's disease)
Parasites
Sclerosing cholangitis
Chronic pancreatitis
AIDS
Mirizzi's syndrome
Oriental cholangiohepatitis
Sump syndrome

cholangitis. A small proportion with severe toxic cholangitis may present with leukopaenia.

- Liver function tests – see above.
- Amylase – mild elevations of amylase are seen in >35% with cholangitis; 11% may have amylase >1000 IU/L; 15% of patients with cholangitis will have associated pancreatitis.
- Blood cultures – see above. Should be taken before commencing antibiotic therapy.
- Coagulation screen – coagulopathy is usually present.

- Abdominal *x* ray – usually unrewarding. In a few patients, calcified gallstones may be seen or gas may be visible in the biliary tree or portal venous system.
- Abdominal ultrasound – see above.
- CT abdomen – may provide additional information about the site and cause of obstruction.
- ERCP – see above.
- PTC – see above.

Management of cholangitis (see Figure 26.1)

Intravenous fluids

Nil by mouth

Intensive care monitoring

Consider invasive monitoring including central venous pressure, urinary catheter, arterial catheter, Swan-Ganz catheter if the patient is in toxic shock.

Coagulation

Correct coagulation with vitamin K or fresh frozen plasma.

Antibiotics

- See Table 26.1 for likely organisms.
- The following regimens are suggested first line therapies until cultures suggest otherwise. They are to be given for 7 days or until biliary decompression is achieved:
  - Ciprofloxacin 500 mg bd orally or 400 mg bd iv
  - Third generation cephalosporin (e.g. cefotaxime 1 or 2 g tid iv) plus metronidazole 500 mg tid iv.
  - Piperacillin 100–150 mg/kg daily in divided doses.
- Most patients will respond to appropriate antibiotics and supportive treatment, allowing a semielective approach to biliary

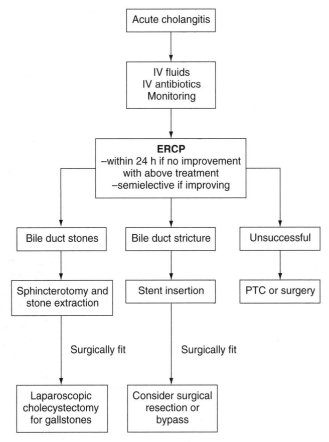

Figure 26.1 Management of a patient with acute cholangitis.

decompression. Failure to respond to antibiotics and intravenous fluids within 24 h is an indication for emergency biliary decompression.

ERCP

- Emergency ERCP is the treatment of choice for patients presenting with severe cholangitis, i.e. with shock and mental confusion, as well as for those patients not responding within 24 h to conservative treatment.
- Endoscopic decompression with sphincterotomy and stone extraction for bile duct stones or stent insertion for strictures,

can be performed successfully in 85–95% of cases with a lower morbidity and mortality compared with percutaneous transhepatic or surgical drainage (see Figure 26.2 and Plates 7–10).

- In a critically ill patient, only brief attempts should be made to remove bile duct stones endoscopically. Decompression of the biliary system with a stent or nasobiliary drain can temporize matters such that subsequent attempts at endoscopic stone removal can be performed safely on a semi-elective basis. Moreover these drainage procedures can be performed without sphincterotomy thus avoiding the risk of haemorrhage due to coagulopathy which frequently accompanies severe cholangitis (see Plate 11).

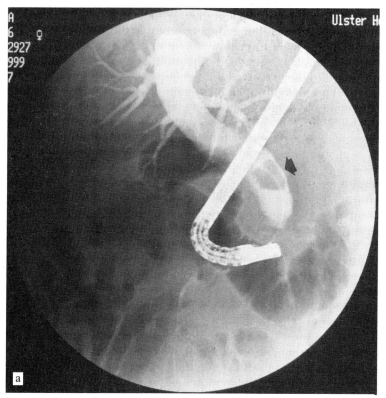

Figure 26.2 (a) ERCP cholangiogram showing a stone in a bile duct (arrowed).

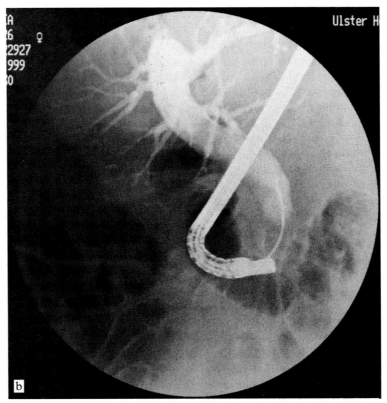

Figure 26.2 (continued) (b) Following sphincterotomy, the stone is extracted and the duct is clear afterwards.

Surgery

- Emergency surgery should be reserved for those in whom endoscopic therapy fails as surgery is associated with a morbidity and mortality of 10–50% depending on the severity of illness and presence of other illnesses. In the emergency situation, surgical decompression of the bile duct is achieved by T-tube drainage, following exploration and extraction of stones. Cholecystectomy should be performed at the same time if the patient is stable or cholecystostomy in an unstable patient.
- In an elective situation, the options include:
  - ERCP with endoscopic sphincterotomy and stone extraction followed by laparoscopic cholecystectomy

- ERCP and leaving the gallbladder *in situ* if the patient is elderly or unfit for surgery
- open cholecystectomy and exploration of the bile duct.

PTC (Percutaneous transhepatic cholangiography)

- Percutaneous transhepatic biliary drainage is usually performed as a temporary measure pending definitive treatment.
- Malignant obstruction can be managed by percutaneous insertion of an internal biliary stent.
- In a few instances, percutaneous access can be used to eliminate biliary stones either by extration using a basket or by chemical dissolution using methyl tertbutyl ether infused down the catheter.
- Complications include bile leak and haemorrhage and can occur in up to 30%.

Further reading

1 Lai ECS, Mok FPT, Tan ESY, *et al.* Endoscopic biliary drainage for severe acute cholangitis. *N Engl J Med* 1992;**326**:1582–6.
2 Lai ECS, Tam PC, Paterson IA, *et al.* Emergency surgery for severe acute cholangitis: the high risk patient. *Ann Surg* 1990;**211**:55–9.
3 Pessa ME, Hawkins IF, Vogel SB. The treatment of acute cholangitis. Percutaneous transhepatic biliary drainage before definitive therapy. *Ann Surg* 1987;**205**:389–92.
4 Speer AG, Cotton PB, Russell RCG, Mason RR, Hatfield AR. Randomised trial of endoscopic versus percutaneous stent insertion in malignant obstructive jaundice. *Lancet* 1987;**ii**:57–62.

27 Variceal haemorrhage

Natural history

Fifty per cent of patients with cirrhosis will bleed from oesophageal varices at some time in their lives. The risk of bleeding from varices (Plate 12) is related to increased portal pressure (> 12 mm Hg), large varices, red colour signs (e.g. cherry red spots, red wale markings, haematocystic spots, diffuse redness of varix), cutaneous vascular spiders and Child's classification.

When bleeding occurs, the mortality is approximately 25–50% with rebleeding and liver failure as the usual cause of death. Seventy per cent will stop bleeding spontaneously but 30–40% will rebleed within 3–4 days and 60% within 7 days. The risk of mortality is highest in the first days to weeks after the variceal bleed and returns to baseline by 3–4 months. Thus therapeutic interventions should be undertaken as early as possible.

History and examination

Please see Chapter 3. Specifically, look for signs of chronic liver disease – jaundice; spider naevis; palmar erythema, gynaecomastia, ascites, encephalopathy; hepatosplenomegaly.

Investigations

- Check full blood picture, cross-match > 6 units, urea and electrolytes, liver function tests, coagulation screen, albumin, alpha-fetoprotein, hepatitis serology, auto-antibody screen.
- When the patient is stabilised, arrange ultrasound scan to look for evidence of cirrhosis, portal hypertension or hepatoma.

Management of acute variceal bleed

General measures

- Resuscitate – intravenous access with two wide bore cannulas, use colloid infusion (e.g. Haemacell) or fresh frozen plasma until blood available, blood transfusion. Avoid use of saline.
- Insert urinary catheter to monitor urine output.
- Consider Intensive Care support with haemodynamic monitoring.
- Transfuse with blood until:
  - arterial pressure is more than 80 mm Hg
  - heart rate less than 100 bpm
  - central venous pressure between 5–10 mm Hg
  - haematocrit between 25–30%.
- Corrrect coagulopathy with fresh frozen plasma and/or platelets.

Pharmacotherapy

- Terlipressin (Glypressin) is effective and has been shown in one study to reduce mortality from variceal bleeding if given early.
  Dose is intravenous bolus injection of 1–2 mg every 4–6 h.
- Octreotide – effective in stopping bleed in 70% of cases although has not been shown to reduce mortality. Just as efficacious as balloon tamponade with fewer complications.
  Dose is 50 mcg bolus then 50 mcg per hour as infusion.
- Propranolol or nadolol is effective in preventing rebleeding. The dose is titrated to achieve a 25% reduction in resting heart rate. The initial dose for propranolol is 40 mg bd, increasing to 80 mg bd according to heart rate, maximum 160 mg bd. This is started as soon as the patient is stabilised following their bleed.
- If propranolol or nadolol are not tolerated, nitrates should be considered as an alternative.

Antibiotic prophylaxis

Giving ciprofloxacin (500–750 mg bd orally or 200–400 mg bd IV) or co-amoxiclav (250–500 mg tid orally or 1 g tid iv) as prophylaxis of bacterial infections in those with ascites can reduce mortality.

Balloon tamponade

- Used if terlipressin or octreotide does not stop bleed or endoscopic therapy not available or unsuccessful.
- Effective in 60–90% of cases. Sixty per cent will rebleed on

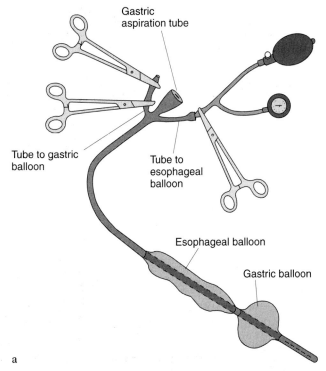

a

Figure 27.1 Placement of balloon tamponade. If the patient is at risk from aspiration e.g. massive harmatemesis in a patient with reduced level of consciousness, endotracheal intubation should be performed first. (a) Modified Sengstaken–Blakemore tube. The tube is passed through the mouth until the 45 cm mark is at incisors (b). Tube position is confirmed by flushing the gastric port with air with auscultation over the stomach or aspiration of gastric contents (c). If there is uncertainty, radiographic confirmation should be obtained. The gastric balloon is then inflated with 250 cc of air, gentle traction applied and tube position confirmed radiographically (d). Approximately 2 pounds of traction is applied to the tube. The gastric and oesophageal ports are also attached to intermittent suction to monitor for further bleeding. The head of the bed is elevated 6–10 inches. Bleeding can often be controlled with inflation of the gastric balloon alone. If bleeding continues, the oesophageal balloon is inflated to a pressure of 25–45 mm Hg. This balloon should not be inflated for more than 24 h.

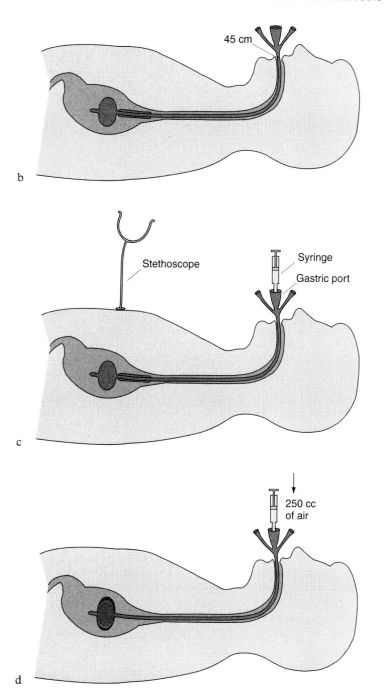

45 cm

b

Stethoscope

Syringe

Gastric port

c

250 cc
of air

d

deflation of balloon. Side effects occur in 10–30%. It is only a temporizing measure until definitive therapy can be instituted.
- Method of placing this is described in Figure 27.1(a)–(d).
- These should NOT be used without first confirming endoscopically that bleeding is variceal in nature. The exception is when a cirrhotic patient presents with a major haemorrhage and is too unstable to undergo endoscopy.

Endoscopic therapy

- Endoscopy should be performed as soon as possible; within 24 h if patient has stopped bleeding or immediately if patient continues to bleed.
- If there is severe ongoing bleeding despite pharmacological therapy, placement of an endotracheal tube to protect the airway from aspiration should be considered.
- In active bleeding, band ligation and sclerotherapy are undertaken. Both achieve haemostasis in 70–90% of cases.
- Band ligation is superior to sclerotherapy in chronic therapy of varices (Figure 27.2). Band ligation has fewer complications, may be associated with lower mortality, requires fewer sessions and rebleeding rate is lower.
- After stopping the bleed, endoscopy should be repeated in 1–3 weeks.

Transjugular intrahepatic portosystemic shunting (TIPS)

- A radiological procedure which decompresses the portal venous circulation by creating a portal to systemic shunt within the liver parenchyma using an expandible stent.
- It is effective in controlling bleed 96–100% of cases with complication rate of 10–25%.
- Hepatic encephalopathy occurs in 15–25% of cases but is severe in only 3–5%.
- It is considered if pharmacologic and endoscopic therapy fails.
- It is particularly useful for treatment of gastric varices.

Surgery

- Oesophageal transection was found to be more effective than sclerotherapy in controlling initial haemorrhage in a randomised study but there was no difference in mortality.
- In acute bleed, emergency shunt surgery has a mortality of 50–80%.
- Transection or shunt surgery (distal splenorenal shunt or

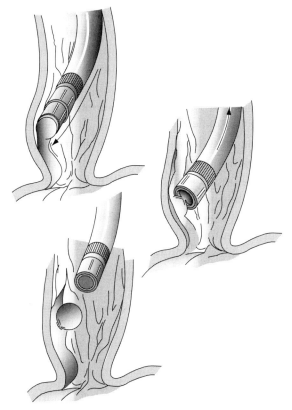

Figure 27.2 Endoscopic band ligation utilises the application of a small suction chamber to an endoscope tip. This allows the varix to be pulled into the stretched band. A trigger device then releases the band around the varix base causing subsequent necrosis and scarring (with permission from Elta GH. Approach to patient with gross gastrointestinal bleeding. *Textbook of Gastroenterology,* 2nd ed, Yamada T (ed), JB Lippincott Co., Philadelphia, 1995.

mesocaval shunt) is considered if pharmacologic and endoscopic therapy fails.

- In preventing bleeding, shunt surgery has no advantage over sclerotherapy.

Liver transplantation

Urgent liver transplantation for acute variceal bleeding is not practical. The greatest benefit of transplantation is for Child's Grade C patients who have had successful control of variceal

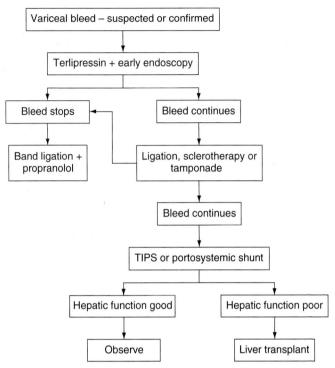

Figure 27.3 Algorithm for the management of an acute variceal haemorrhage.

bleeding by the usual treatment measures and then undergo elective transplantation.

Failure of therapy

- 10% of patients will fail initial pharmacologic and endoscopic therapy.
- For the choice of therapeutic options: TIPS, surgery or liver transplantation, see Figure 27.3.
- Consider non-oesophageal sites of haemorrhage, e.g. gastric varices, portal hypertensive gastropathy or ectopic varices. Patients with cirrhosis may also bleed from causes unrelated to portal hypertension, e.g. duodenal ulcer.

Treatment of hepatic encephalopathy, renal failure

Please see Chapter 28.

Further reading

1 Burroughs AK, Planas R, Svoboda P. Optimizing emergency care of upper gastrointestinal bleeding in cirrhotic patients. *Scand J Gastroenterol Suppl* 1998;**226**:14–24

2 Cello JP, Grendell JH, Crass RA, *et al.* Endoscopic sclerotherapy versus portacaval shunt in patients with severe cirrhosis and acute variceal haemorrhage. *N Engl J Med* 1987;**316**:1589–600.

3 D'Amico G, Pagliaro L, Bosch J. The treatment of portal hypertension: a meta-analytic review. *Hepatology* 1995;**22**:332–54.

4 Ewaga H, Keefe EB, Dort J, *et al.* Liver transplantation for uncontrollable variceal bleeding. *Am J Gastroenterol* 1994;**89**:1823–6.

5 Jalan R, Hayes PC. UK guidelines on the management of variceal haemorrhage in cirrhotic patients. *Gut* 2000;**46** (suppl III): iii1–iii15.

6 Levacher S, Letoumelin P, Pateron D, Blaise M, Lapandry C, Pourriat JL. Early administration of terlipressin plus glyceryl trinitrate to control active upper gastrointestinal bleeding in cirrhotic patients. *Lancet* 1995;**346**(8979):865–8.

7 Shiffman ML, Jeffers L, Hoofnagle JH, *et al.* The role of transjugular intrahepatic portosystemic shunt for therapy of portal hypertension and its complications: a conference sponsored by the national digestive disease advisory board. *Hepatology* 1995;**22**:1591–7.

8 Stiegmann GV, Goff JS, Michaletz-Onody PA, *et al.* Endoscopic sclerotherapy as compared with endoscopic ligation for bleeding esophageal varices. *N Engl J Med* 1992;**326**:1527–32.

9 Sung JJY, Chung SCS, Lei CW, *et al.* Octreotide infusion or emergency sclerotherapy for variceal haemorrhage. *Lancet* 1993;**141**:637–41.

28 Acute liver failure

Introduction

Fulminant hepatic failure (FHF) is defined as "a potentially reversible condition, the consequence of severe liver injury, with onset of encephalopathy within 8 weeks of the appearance of the first symptoms and in the absence of pre-existing liver disease".

In the UK, the broadly accepted classification is:

- Hyperacute- with jaundice < 7 days the onset of encephalopathy
- acute-with jaundice 8–28 days before onset
- subacute-jaundice for 4–12 weeks before onset.

Aetiology

The main causes of FHF are infections , drugs or toxins. A proportion of cases are due to miscellaneous or idiosyncratic causes (Table 28.1).

Table 28.1 Causes of fulminant hepatic failure.

Infections	Drugs/toxins	Miscellaneous
Viral	Parcetamol	Hepatic hypoperfusion
Bacterial	Mushrooms	Malignancy
Parasitic	Carbon tetrachloride*	Wilson's disease
	Anti-TB drugs*	Acute fatty liver of pregnancy
	Sulphonamides*	Reye's syndrome
	NSAIDs*	Trauma
	Ketoconazole*	Liver graft rejection
	Tricyclics*	

*Idiosyncratic drug reaction.

Infectious causes

On a worldwide basis viral hepatitis A,B,D and E are the commonest causes of FHF. Of the viral hepatitides, Hep B is the commonest single cause with or without Hep D. Hep E is usually encountered in the Indian sub-continent, the Middle East and Mexico. Hep C and G are not recognised as causes of acute liver failure.

Other less commonly encountered viral causes include Coxsackie, Herpes simplex, Epstein-Barr, Cytomegalovirus, adenovirus and varicella-zoster.

Tuberculosis, *Coxiella burneti* and typhoid have all been reported as possible bacterial causes while amoebiasis and malaria are tropical parasitic causes.

Drugs and toxins

Paracetamol toxicity is dose dependent (see below) with malnourished individuals and alcoholic patients with liver enzyme induction at highest risk. The toxic mushroom *Amanita phalloides* is mostly commonly encountered as a cause in central Europe and the Western USA. Drugs such as ketoconazole, for example, may lead to FHF .

Miscellaneous causes

In the Budd–Chiari syndrome, acute obstruction of the hepatic veins leads to hepatocyte ischaemia and centrilobular necrosis. Veno-occlusive disease is seen in 10–20% of patients after chemotherapy and radiotherapy associated with bone marrow transplantation. General hypoperfusion as in cases of acute blood loss or cardiogenic shock can be followed by massive liver cell necrosis.

Massive liver infiltration as a consequence of terminal metastatic carcinoma or lymphoma may present in the late stages with FHF.

Wilson's disease is an inherited disorder of copper transportation where high tissue copper levels lead to cirrhosis proceeding in some cases to FHF which is the presenting syndrome in young adults.

Assessment

The diagnosis of FHF may be difficult or delayed in the early stages because there is no pre-existing history of chronic liver disease. It should be suspected in any patient who is drowsy (see below), jaundiced and who has a history of possible recent viral hepatitis, drug usage or possible overdose. The clinical features common to all cases are:

- Encephalopathy – the patient with FHF will invariably exhibit one of the stages of acute hepatic encephalopathy outlined below in Table 28.2.
- Asterixis may be absent due to the rapid onset of coma and jaundice may not be overt.
- Cerebral oedema – this is responsible for over 50% of all deaths due to FHF and is usually seen in grade 3 and 4 encephalopathy. Early signs are sluggish pupillary response, increased muscle tone and decerebrate posturing in the late stages.
- Metabolic disorders:
  Hypoglycaemia – this is a serious complication which will lead to rapid onset of coma. It is due to an inability of the necrotic liver to mobilise glycogen stores.
  Hyponatraemia – there is water retention by the kidney and a serum Na of less than 120 mmol/l will contribute to encephalopathy.
  Hypokalaemia – this is frequently found before renal impairment occurs and may be related to hyperaldosteronism and increased plasma insulin levels.
  Hypocalcaemia – serum calcium levels may fall. Total serum calcium must be corrected for low serum albumin levels.
  Hypomagnesaemia – levels should be assessed along with calcium.

Table 28.2 Grading of encephalopathy.

Grade 0	Normal
Subclinical	Abnormal psychometric tests
Grade 1	Euphoria or depression, disturbed sleep
	May have asterixis, impaired drawing
Grade 2	Drowsy, grossly impaired calculation
Grade 3	Confusion, disorientation, drowsy and somnolent but arousable, asterixis
Grade 4	Deep coma, unresponsive to stimulae

Hypophosphataemia – this is commonly seen particularly in paracetamol poisoning and it may contribute to respiratory failure.

Acid/base disturbance – FHF results in the accumulation of organic anions e.g. pyruvate, acetoacetate and succinate. This leads to a metabolic acidosis in 5% of cases and has been reported in up to 30% of paracetamol cases. In most cases of FHF a metabolic alkalosis results from a combination of factors.

- Coagulopathy – the factors contributing to this complication are outlined in Table 28.3.

  Disseminated intravascular coagulation is often present at low grade as manifested by increased fibrin degradation products.

- Involvement of other systems:

  Renal failure – this occurs early in about 30% of all cases and 75% of paracetamol cases. Hepatorenal syndrome is the most important cause renal failure and results in oliguria despite unremarkable urinary sediment and histologically normal kidneys.

  Cardiovascular disorders – hypotension is often present in FHF due to generalised vasodilatation and results in a relative hypovolaemia. This development may be exacerbated by sepsis, bleeding and hypoxia.

  Respiratory failure – pulmonary oedema occurs in 33% of patients and Adult Respiratory Distress syndrome is seen in patients in grade 4 coma.

- Infection – The incidence of bacteraemia in FHF is 20–40% and bacterial infection is a common cause of morbidity and mortality. The most commonly isolated organisms are *Staph aureus*, *E. coli* and *Pseudomonas aeruginosa*.

  Fungal sepsis is common due to impaired immune defences.

Table 28.3 Coagulopathy factors in FHF.

Blood investigation	Result
Platelets	Decreased
INR	Prolonged
PTT	Prolonged
Fibrinogen	Decreased
AT III	Decreased
Plasminogen	Decreased

Examination

The following are important clinical signs in the initial assessment:

- Fever, jaundice, sweating, tachycardia.
- Presence of foetor, Kayser–Fleischer rings in cornea.
- Tachypnoea, crepitations at lung bases.
- Hypotension.
- Hepatomegaly or signs of small liver with chronic stigmata of liver disease.
- Ascites.
- Pregnancy.
- Splenomegaly.
- Tender enlarged liver ? Due to viral hepatitis.
- Grade of encephalopathy (see above).

Investigations

Investigations should:

1 Establish the cause – paracetamol levels, viral hepatitis screen and HBV DNA levels with hepatitis D antibody, HSV serology; CMV IgM, EBV antibody titres, serum cearuloplasmin to rule out Wilson's disease.

   Liver ultrasound to detect Budd–Chiari, neoplasm and ascites/splenomegaly.
2 Confirm the diagnosis – serum transaminases, alkaline phosphatase, bilirubin, blood glucose.
3 Predict prognosis and complications – coagulation screen, urea and electrolytes, urinary electrolytes, ECG, chest x ray.

The laboratory abnormalities associated with FHF are shown in Table 28.4

Management

General

There are three dominant clinical problems associated with FHF which govern the subsequent management.

- Neurological – these include encephalopathy and raised intracranial pressure (see above), neurohypoxaemia and seizure activity.
- Haemodynamic instability.
- Infection.

Table 28.4 Laboratory abnormalities in FHF.

Investigation	Result
FBC	Decreased PCV Normal or increased WBCC Low platelets
U&E	Decreased Na^+ Decreased K^+ Decreased HCO_3^- Decreased or normal glucose
Liver function	Slight to markedly increased transaminases Low to slightly increased alk. phosphatase Mild to markedly increased bilirubin Decreased albumin
Arterial blood gas	Normal or decreased pH Normal or low pO_2 Variable pCO_2 Elevated ammonia

The general primary aims are to provide full support and clinical monitoring and to identify those patients who will benefit from liver transplantation as soon as possible after the diagnosis is made.

All patients with FHF should be admitted or transferred to an HDU environment, in a centre with a hepatology unit with a liver transplant service.

Treatment of specific complications

Hepatic encephalopathy

- The grade of encephalopathy (see above) should be assessed. Benzodiazepines in particular should be avoided along with narcotics. Lactulose 30 ml qds combined with neomycin 2–4 g orally for 3 days may delay progression of coma. If possible the patient's colon should be cleared daily and the aim is to produce two or three soft stools daily with the lactulose. Metronidazole 400 mg bd or vancomycin 1000 mg bd have also been used although the former may cause nausea. The implementation of a restricted protein diet may worsen pre-existing nutritional deficiencies and dietary supplementation with branch-chained amino acids 1–1·2 g/kg/day has been used with mixed success.

- Raised intra-cranial pressure (ICP) and its signs are discussed above. The patient should be intubated and hyperventilated to reduce CO_2 levels below 30 mm Hg. Mannitol should be given as a single iv bolus of 0·3–0·5 mg/kg usually 100 ml of a 20% solution. Seizures should be treated with short-acting benzo-diazepines as they occur. Auditory and tactile stimuli should be minimised.

Haemodynamic instability

The patient's blood pressure requires close monitoring. The use of crystalloid infusions to treat hypotension can be associated with pulmonary oedema and pulmonary artery wedge pressure moni-toring will help predict impending fluid overload.

Infection

Frequent surveillance of blood, urine and sputum for bacteria and fungi as well as meticulous attention to asepsis for iv line care are essential.

Other complications

Metabolic

Electrolyte, glucose and acid/base status requires close monitor-ing. Metabolic acidosis may require iv bicarbonate or even dialysis. Hypoglycaemia requires iv dextrose to maintain plasma glucose levels above 3·5 mmol/l.

Renal failure

If renal failure develops, haemodialysis may be required in some patients to treat uraemia, fluid overload and acid/base imbalance.

Liver transplantation

This operation is now widely accepted as life-saving in patients with FHF. About 50% of patients with FHF unrelated to parac-etamol damage undergo orthotopic liver transplantation with survival rates of up to 93%. Data from King's Liver Unit suggest that the best prognosis is in acute fatty liver of pregnancy. In cases of viral hepatitis, non-ABCD had the worst prognosis. The indications for referral in paracetamol overdose is detailed in Chapter 29.

Extracorporeal liver support

Several studies have reported benefit from the use of a perfused column of porcine hepatocytes used as a supportive "bridge" until a transplant can be arranged. All of these devices are in various stages of development but may become standard therapies to reduce complications and even allow the diseased liver to recover from the initial damage.

Further reading

1   O'Grady JG, SChalm S, Williams R. Acute liver failure: redefining the syndromes. *Lancet* 1993;**342**:273–5.
2   Williams R, Gimson AES. Intensive liver care and management of acute liver failure. *Dig Dis Sci* 1991;**36**:820–6.

29 Paracetamol toxicity

Introduction

Paracetamol is widely used as a simple analgesic. In overdose as little as 20–30 tablets (10–15 g) may lead to severe liver damage and fulminant hepatic failure. The mechanism of damage is related to conjugation of the electrophilic metabolite of the drug with hepatic glutathione. When available glutathione is used up, the toxic metabolites arylate essential nucleophilic macromolecules which cause hepatic cell necrosis.

Management

Assessment

Within 2–3 h of the initial ingestion, the patient may develop nausea and vomiting but these symptoms settle within 24 h in most cases. If the patient is untreated and the dose is significant, after 48 h jaundice may develop followed by the signs of fulminant hepatic failure (see Chapter 28).

Hepatic histology in severe cases shows centrizonal necrosis and reticulin collapse.

Treatment

- In all cases patients should be referred to hospital as an emergency. This is appropriate even if the patient has vomited a quantity of the drug .
- Patients particularly at high risk are:
    - those on enzyme–inducing drugs e.g. carbamazipine, phenobarbitone, rifampicin.
    - patients with a high alcohol intake.
    - malnourished patients.

- Gastric lavage should be carried out if the overdose has been ingested in the past 2 h.
- Plasma paracetamol level should be related to time of ingestion on a paracetamol treatment graph (see Figure 29.1) provided the time from ingestion is not less than 4 h as levels may be misleading. Those with paracetamol levels above the normal treatment line should be treated with intravenous acetylcysteine (Parvolex) in glucose 5% initially 150 mg/kg in 200 ml over 15 min followed by 50 mg/kg in 500 ml over 4 h, then 100 mg/kg in 1000 ml over 16 h.
- Provided the overdose has been taken within 10–12 h an alternative therapy is to give oral methionine 2·5 g initially, followed by three further doses of methionine at 4 h intervals
- In the high risk patient group, toxicity may develop at lower plasma paracetamol levels and should be treated if levels are above the high risk line (Figure 29.1)
- If there is any doubt about the time from ingestion and the levels, the patient should be treated.

Progressive liver failure

Unfortunately, due to a delay in notification or diagnosis, some patients progress to show signs of fulminant hepatic failure. The clinical details have been described in the chapter on FHF. Laboratory tests will show:

- Raised serum creatinine.
- Massively elevated liver transaminases >1000.
- Coagulopathy with prothrombin time > 30 s.
- Arterial pH < 7·3.
- Often hyopglycaemia blood glucose < 3·5 mmol/l.

In these cases, the patient should be discussed with a specialist liver unit and preparations made for transfer. King's College Hospital's Liver Unit has defined helpful guidelines for this purpose (Table 29.1)

N-acetylcysteine in late diagnosis

This antidote can be given up to 36 h after ingestion and appears to have a beneficial effect with a lower incidence of cerebral oedema, and less haemodynamic instability.

Liver transplant

Some patients will require hepatic transplantation.

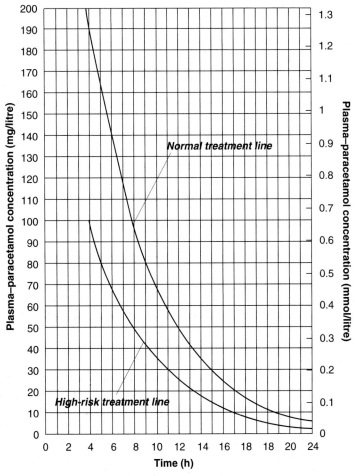

Figure 29.1 Plasma paracetamol treatment graphs (source: *BNF*, 1998).

Table 29.1 King's College Hospital Liver Unit guidelines for referral after paracetamol OD.

Day 2	Day 3	Day 4
Art pH < 7.3	Art pH < 7.3	
INR >3.0	INR >4.5	Rise in INR
Oliguria	Oliguria	Oliguria
Creat >200	Creat > 200	Creat >300
Hypogycaemia	Encephalopathy	Encephalopathy

30 Ascites

Introduction

The term ascites means the accumulation of free fluid within the peritoneal cavity and becomes clinically evident when 1 l is present. It is the most common presentation of decompensated cirrhosis and implies a poor prognosis. It may present as an acute GI emergency as a distended painful abdomen or more rarely associated with the development of spontaneous bacterial peritonitis.

Aetiology

In cirrhosis, portal hypertension is associated with low arterial pressure and peripheral resistance which in turn stimulates endogenous vasoconstrictor systems. The kidney retains sodium and water and the plasma volume is expanded. As the underlying liver disease progresses, splanchnic arteriolar vasodilatation is increased and can no longer be compensated for because the retained fluid is sequestered in the peritoneal space.

The time-honoured classification of ascites into transudate and exudate based on the protein content has now been questioned as a recent study showed that 56% of patients were able to be correctly diagnosed using this method. A better classification measures the ascitic protein level and subtracts it from the serum albumin level – the serum-ascites gradient.

Serum albumin minus ascitic albumin level in g/dl:
transudate is $>1\cdot1$ g/dl
exudate is $<1\cdot1$ g/dl.

Based on this measurement, Runyon has classified the causes of ascites as follows.

Related to portal hypertension (gradient>1.1 g/dl)

- cirrhosis
- alcoholic hepatitis
- cardiac ascites
- massive liver metastasis
- fulminant hepatic failure
- Budd–Chiari syndrome
- portal vein thrombosis
- veno-occlusive disease
- fatty liver of pregnancy
- myxoedema.

Unrelated to portal hypertension (gradient < 1·1 g/dl)

- peritoneal carcinomatosis
- TB
- pancreatic ascites
- biliary ascites
- nephrotic syndrome
- serositis in connective tissue diseases

History

- The patient will usually complain of a noticeable increase in abdominal girth on a possible background of chronic liver disease.
- Some patients may report ankle swelling and dyspnoea.
- It is important to enquire about alcohol intake and past history of cardio-respiratory disease and renal disease.

Examination

On clinical examination the classical signs of ascites will often be apparent.

- Bulging flanks or generally distended abdomen.
- Dullness to percussion in the flanks with "shifting dullness".
- The presence of a fluid wave or "thrill".

Investigations

- If the clinical impression is uncertain, abdominal ultrasound can accurately establish the presence of as little as 100 ml of fluid as well as providing useful information on the liver, spleen, pancreas and ovaries.

- In most patients,especially at first presentation, a diagnostic paracentesis should be carried out. This is performed under strict sterile conditions, by passing an intra-muscular needle into the left lower abdominal quadrant under local anaesthetic.

  The following data should be obtained:
  - routine cell count
  - albumin
  - culture
  - total protein
  - cytology
  - in some cases-amylase, TB culture, LDH and glucose.

  The main ascitic fluid findings are shown in Table 30.1. Complications of diagnostic paracenteseis have been reported. These include:
  - bowel perforation
  - abdominal wall haematoma
  - puncture of aberrant varicosities
  - introduction of infection leading to ascites
  - leakage.

  The findings in spontaneous bacterial peritonitis are discussed below.

Treatment

- Bedrest increases glomerular filtration rate.
- Dietary sodium should be restricted to 2 g/day.
- If tolerated restrict oral fluids to 1200–1500 ml/day.
- Start oral spironolactone 100 mg daily.
- If no response after 5 days add frusemide 40 mg daily.

Table 30.1

Condition	Albumin (g/dl)	WBCs/ml	RBCs/ml	Ascites-albumin gradient (g/dl)
Cirrhosis	<2·5	300–500	<1000	>1·1
Hepatoma	<2·5	300–500	1000–50000	>1·1
Carcinomatosis	>2·5	Variable	usually < 1000	<1·1
Cardiogenic	>2·5–3·0	300–500	< 1000	>1·1

- Increase the doses stepwise to spironolactone 400 mg and frusemide 160 mg daily.
- Monitor the patients' urinary output and body weight seeking a weight loss of 500g–1kg per day.
- Monitor urea and electrolytes during diuretic phase.
- Watch for signs of hepatic encephalopathy.

Management of refractory ascites

This is defined as the group of patients who fail to achieve negative sodium balance or develop complications of the medical therapy. They constitute 10% of all cases of ascites. Treatment options for these patients are:
- Repeated therapeutic paracentesis.
- Peritoneovenous shunting.
- Transjugular intrahepatic portosystemic shunt (TIPS).
- Extracorporeal ultrafiltration of ascitic fluid with reinfusion.
- Liver transplant.

Therapeutic paracentesis

This has been reported and widely used and is safe enough to perform as a daycase procedure. Up to 10 l of ascitic fluid can be removed, using a 16 ga needle, in 30–60 min. The procedure can be repeated until a more definitive procedure is indicated but is a useful palliative in patients where surgical management is contraindicated. Some centres have suggested that the patients should be given plasma volume expanders in the form of albumin or Dextran infusion. However, this has not been shown to decrease mortality or the incidence of hepato-renal syndrome.

Peritoneo-venous shunting

This is indicated if a patient cannot tolerate repeat paracentesis. The operation has been associated with a high complication rate. The shunts block after 1 year in about 50% of patients. Hepatic encephalopathy has been reported in 15%, severe bacterial infection in 6% and disseminated intravascular coagulation in 6%. It is now only indicated in patients unfit for liver transplant or who have multiple abdominal scars making repeated paracentesis impossible.

TIPS

This technique involves the placement of an expandable stent between the portal vein and the hepatic vein. Reports of a 70%

success rate in ascites relief have been published. The technique has a 25% morbidity and is associated with intra abdominal bleeding and encephalopathy. It is also useful in refractory oesophageal variceal bleeding. It may act as a "bridge" procedure in patients awaiting liver transplantation.

Further reading

1 Akriviadis E, Runyon BA. Ascites and acute hemoperitoneum. In: Taylor M, ed. *Gastrointestinal emergencies.* Baltimore: Williams and Wilkins, 1997: 473–81
2 Runyon BA, Reynolds TB. Approach to the patient with ascites. In: Yamada T, Alpers D, Owyang C, Powell D, Silverstein F, eds. *Textbook of gastroenterology.* New York: Lippincott, 1991: 846–64.

31 Spontaneous bacterial peritonitis

Introduction

This condition is defined as a bacterial infection of ascitic fluid which is not associated with an identifiable source of intra-abdominal sepsis. It has been reported that over 25% of ascitic patients will develop an episode of SBP within the first year after diagnosis.

Unfortunately the 5 year survival of SBP survivors is only of the order of 20%, most deaths due to recurrent SBP or the underlying liver disease. Other major complications leading to death are septicaemia, hepatorenal syndrome, GI bleeding and liver failure.

Aetiology

In the absence of ascites SBP is rare. The source of infection appears to be from the gut lumen but the access route is unclear.

Patients with advanced liver disease are especially prone to bacteraemia and have impaired immunity with loss of first pass clearing of bacteria by the liver.

History and examination

The signs and symptoms of SBP may be identical to those of secondary peritonitis. In order of incidence they are listed below:

- jaundice
- pyrexia
- abdominal pain
- hepatic encephalopathy
- abdominal tenderness
- rebound tenderness

- diminished or absent bowel sound
- diarrhoea
- hypotension
- hypothermia.

Investigations

The most important investigations in suspected cases is a diagnostic paracentesis,when the fluid should be sent for cell count, culture, and cytology, serum biochemistry and blood cultures.

The findings in the ascitic fluid are summarised in Table 31.1.

The common bacteria isolated from the ascitic fluid are *E. coli*, *Klebsiella pneumoniae*, *Strep pneumoniae* and *Grp D streptococcus*. Positive blood cultures have been reported in 54% of patients with the majority reporting the same organism isolated in the ascitic fluid.

Additional investigations

If the ascitic and blood investigations are equivocal or suggest a possible Secondary Peritonitis, the patient should have a plain abdominal radiograph performed. Exclude an intra-abdominal perforation and an ultrasound/CT scan to rule out a liver or pelvic abscess.

Treatment

Untreated or inappropriately treated SBP is associated with a high mortality of 30–40%.

A high degree of clinical suspicion is required combined with a prompt diagnostic paracentesis.

Table 31.1 Ascites fluid results in SBP and secondary peritonitis.

	SBP	Secondary
Cloudy appearance	Seen in 80%	Seen in 90%
Absolute PMNs	Av 6 000	Av 8 000
pH	Reduced in 60–70%	Reduced > 70%
Glucose	Reduced in 10%	Reduced in 90%
LDH > serum conc	Mean 20%	Mean 90%
Organisms	Monomicrobial	Polymicrobial

Source: Hoefs JC, Jonas G. Spontaneous bacterial peritonitis. In: Taylor MB, ed. *Gastrointestinal emergencies*. Baltimore: Williams & Wilkins, 1997: 485.

Antibiotic treatment should be started.

- If the clinical picture suggests SBP despite a normal ascitic neutrophil count.
- The neutrophil count >250/cu mm even if other clinical evidence is lacking.

Treatment with empirically chosen antibiotics should be started before ascitic and/or blood culture results are available. The following are important points.

- Anaerobic organisms are uncommon in SBP and do not require specific coverage.
- Gentamicin should be avoided in cirrhotic patients.
- Third generation cephalosporins, e.g. cefotaxime 750 mg iv every 6 h is recommended first line therapy.
- Usually treatment should be continued for 10–14 days.

In some patients the neutrophil count will be greater than $250/mm^3$ but culture will be negative. This situation has been called culture negative neutrocytic ascites (CNNA). This variant should be treated identically to a culture positive case.

32 Alcoholic hepatitis

Introduction

Although this condition is usually associated with a heavy regular alcohol intake, mild forms may occur associated with deranged liver enzymes and a macrocytosis. Modest doses of paracetamol may precipitate an attack in an alcoholic because of induction of microsomal metabolism leading to a build-up of toxic metabolites.

Aetiology/mechanisms of liver injury

Alcohol must be oxidised to acetaldehyde in the cytosol of the liver cell by the action of ADH. Fatty acids accumulates and may lead to fatty liver. The acetaldehyde is broken down further to acetate by the action of aldehyde dehydrogenase. Around 10–15% of alcohol is metabolised by a P450 oxidising system which is inducible by alcohol and drugs increasing the risk of enhanced toxic metabolites during the degradation of potentially hepatotoxic drugs.

The toxic effects of acetaldehyde include interference with the mitochondrial transport chain, increased collagen synthesis and the stimulation of neutrophils to produce superoxides.

Immunological mechanisms account for the finding of elevation of serum immunoglobulin levels and evidence of CD4 and CD8-expressing lymphocytes in advanced alcoholic hepatitis. In severely ill patients, endotoxin is often detected in the peripheral blood which in turn leads to the release of cytokines IL1, IL2, and TNF in non-parenchymal cells. It has been suggested that the stimulus for cytokine production is related to alcohol-induced liver injury. The biological effects of cytokines are similar to those seen in advanced liver disease – fever, muscle wasting, neutrophilia, decreased bile flow and shock.

History

Florid acute alcoholic hepatitis is rare and usually presents as a spectrum of severity:

- mild alcoholic hepatitis, relatively asymptomatic
- fatty liver
- severe alcoholic hepatitis, often with underlying cirrhosis.

Patients in the mild category may feel well and the diagnosis will only be made on the basis of a liver biopsy performed because of persistently abnormal liver function tests.

A careful alcohol history, accompanied by the CAGE questionnare:

- C = felt need to cut do down intake?
- A = annoyed at even the suggestion of a problem?
- G = guilty of drinking to excess?
- E = drink in morning?

One point is scored for each positive response and scores of > 2 = alcohol problems.

In the patient with fatty liver, there may be fatigue and mild pyrexia. Nausea and vomiting may be present associated with vague upper abdominal pain. The severe case will complain of anorexia, jaundice and prolonged vomiting. Hepatic decompensation may have been precipitated by an infection, prolonged fasting or paracetamol.

Examination

In severe cases clinical signs are:

- fever
- jaundice
- very enlarged, tender, liver
- arterial murmur over liver in 50%
- vascular skin spiders
- hepatic encephalopathy
- bruising or bleeding gums
- signs of malnutrition and vitamin deficiencies
- low blood pressure
- hyperdynamic circulation
- diarrhoea with steatorrhoea due to inadequate production of bile salts

- shock
- GI haemorrhage.

Investigation

- The results of laboratory investigations in alcoholic hepatitis are shown in Table 32.1.
- In some cases the patient will present with a cholestatic syndrome with deep jaundice, hepatomegaly, raised transaminases and alkaline phosphatase.
- Patients with acute alcoholic pancreatitis have an increased incidence of viral hepatitis markers than the normal population and co-existing viral disease may increase the severity of the underlying liver damage.
- Liver biopsy gives a good idea of prognosis. Unfavourable features are Zone 3 fibrosis and peri-venular sclerosis. Histological cholestasis is also an adverse prognostic indicator. A combination of cirrhosis and alcoholic hepatitis appears to have the worst prognosis.

Treatment

The following are the mainstays of therapy in acute alcoholic hepatitis:

Complete abstinence from alcohol

The rapid development of alcoholic withdrawal

The patient should be sedated with chlordiazepoxide 30 mg tds, gradually reducing. A close watch must be made for the signs of impending encephalopathy. An adequate diet containing 0·5 mg/kg

Table 32.1 Laboratory investigations in acute alcoholic hepatitis.

Investigation	Result
Serum transaminases	Markedly elevated
AST:ALT ratio	>2
IgA	Increased
IgG	Increased
Albumin	Decreased
Potassium	Decreased
Polymorphs	Increased
Platelet function	Decreased

body weight of protein should be provided and increased to 1·0 gm/kg unless hepatic encephalopathy is present. The aim should be to provide a 2000 cal diet with vitamin supplements.

Treat precipitating factors, particularly infection

Corticosteroid therapy

The trial results in this area are controversial with some studies failing to show a beneficial clinical effect of steroids on recovery or biochemical parameters. One multi-centre trial (see further reading) treated patients with either spontaneous encephalopathy or a discriminant function > 32 (calculated by formula 4·6 × increase in PTT in secs + bilirubin) with either placebo or methylprednisolone 30 mg daily and showed a significant improvement in survival in the treated group. A meta-analysis has also shown short term benefits for steroid therapy. At present, steroids are probably most useful for those patients who present with encephalopathy.

Amino acid supplementation

Unfortunately, trials of branched chain amino acid-enhanced diets have failed to show benefit and oral or intravenous amino acid supplementation should be reserved for jaundiced and severely malnourished patients.

Propylthiouracil

Due to the hypermetabolic state which alcohol induces in liver cells, propylthiouracil has been shown to have a beneficial effect on acute alcoholic hepatitis in the animal model and in one clinical trial. However its effects are limited and it is not widely used in this condition.

Liver transplantation

This is the ultimate resort for patients with terminal alcoholic hepatitis with or without cirrhosis. Selection for transplant is confined to patients who are abstinent for 6 months, with Child's Grade C liver disease (bilirubin >100, albumin <30, ascites, encephalopathy and poor nutrition).

Further reading

1 Carithers RL, Herlong HF, Diehl AM, *et al*. Methylprednisolone therapy in patients with severe alcoholic hepatitis. A randomized multi-centre trial. *Ann Intern Med* 1989;**110**:685.
2 Sherlock S. Alcoholic liver disease. *Lancet* 1995; **345**: 227–9.

33 Acute appendicitis

Introduction

Although this is a common gastrointestinal emergency which usually comes under the initial care of GPs then surgeons, the exact pathogenesis is still unclear. The "obstruction" theory states that faecalith impaction in the appendiceal lumen leads to swelling, wall ischaemia and secondary infection. Other workers have argued that obstruction plays no part in the condition and that blood-borne infection is the main cause with obstruction playing a secondary role.

History

The peak incidence of acute appendicitis is in the second decade of life. The main aim of early diagnosis in this condition is to avoid the complication of a perforated appendix with the subsequent development of an abscess or widespread peritonitis. The main clinical features are as follows:

- Abdominal pain which usually begins in the epigastric or peri-umbilical area in 70% of cases and migrates to the right iliac fossa in 50%.
- Anorexia, nausea or vomiting is present in 90%.
- The patient may notice mild dysuria.

Examination

The physical findings are an important pointer to the diagnosis and particular attention should be made to a careful rectal examination to check for pelvic tenderness. The main signs are:

- Fever (in 20%).
- Right iliac fossa tenderness 45–60%.
- Abdominal guarding 10–15%.
- Abdominal mass 10–15%.
- A positive "psoas sign" 10–15% – in this case, with the patient in the supine position, the right knee is flexed and the right hip extended against resistance, the test is positive if pain is felt in the pelvic region.
- Rovsing's sign – palpation of the left lower abdomen produces tenderness on the right side.
- Right sided rectal/pelvic tenderness 45–60% – may be present in other conditions such as pelvic inflammatory disease in women.

Unusual presentations

In cases of retrocaecal appendix, the classic shift of pain from central to right side may be absent, abdominal tenderness is minimal or even absent, guarding is absent and there will be absent rectal tenderness.

In pelvic appendix, the pain shift will be more to the left side, abdominal tenderness and guarding are absent. There may be an urge for the patient to urinate or defaecate and rectal tenderness is present.

The differential diagnosis of acute appendicitis is large and varied (Table 33.1).

Table 33.1 Differential diagnosis of acute appendictis.

Site of pathology	Diagnosis
Unknown	Non-specific abdominal pain
Female reproductive	Pelvic inflammatory disease
	Ovarian cyst
	Ectopic pregnancy
Small bowel	Crohn's Disease
	Ileal perforation
	Meckel diverticulum
	Adenocarcinoma
	Obstruction
Colon	Diverticulitis
	Carcinoma of caecum
Infections	TB
	Yersinia

Investigations

The most commonly requested is the white blood cell count which will be elevated above 10 000 with a shift to the left in 90% of cases. Plain abdominal radiographs may show a dilated loop of small bowel in the right lower quadrant, caecal dilatation, loss of the psoas margin or an appendicolith.

Recently, abdominal ultrasonography and CT scanning have been studied as methods of improving diagnostic accuracy and although they may decrease the negative laparotomy rate by about 5%, they are not universally applicable and generally not accepted as routine investigations.

Treatment

Although there is a negative laparotomy rate of 8–26% in this disease, appendicectomy remains the mainstay of treatment. The appendix can be removed laparoscopically – a technique which has been shown to be safe and effective. The advantage appears to be cost savings due to a lower time spent in hospital. However there is a considerable initial capital outlay on equipment and the ultimate cost effectiveness of "lap appendicectomy" has been questioned.

Treatment of complications of appendicitis

The main complications are:

- *Perforation* – seen in 15–20% of patients aged 6–65 years. Treatment should consist of intravenous antibiotics to cover Gram negative aerobes and anaerobes, intravenous fluids and early operation. Mortality rates in this situation are 0·5–0·9% compared to 0–0·2% in uncomplicated cases.
- *Appendiceal mass* – this is either a phlegmon due to walled off abscess and omentum or inflammation in the absence of an actual abscess. Treatment can be conservative with intravenous fluids and antibiotics until the mass resolves, when an "interval appendicectomy" can be performed. Some surgeons, however, advocate an early surgical approach with good results and no difference in mortality. The assessment of these patients with ultrasound and CT will help to

differentiate the diagnosis from ileo-caecal Crohn's disease or a caecal carcinoma.

- *Infertility* – tubal involvement from a perforated appendix is only avoided by early operative therapy in young females.

34 Intestinal obstruction

with contributions from John Moorehead, Paul Neilly

Introduction

Intestinal obstruction is caused by mechanical blockage (dynamic obstruction) or insufficient peristalsis (adynamic obstruction) and may be partial or complete. The condition is also classified according to the level of obstruction (high/low, small bowel/colon) as the presentation and management may differ significantly. The causes of dynamic and adynamic obstruction are summarised in Tables 34.1 and 34.2.

Table 34.1 Aetiology of dynamic bowel obstruction.

Inside the lumen	Faeces
	Foreign body/bezoar
	Gallstone
	Polyp +/- intussusception
Within the wall	Congenital – atresia, stenosis, Hirschsprung's disease
	Inflammatory stricture – diverticulosis, Crohn's disease, infectious enteritis, radiation, chemical, endometriosis
	Other strictures – ischaemia, anastomotic, neoplastic, haematoma
	Intussusception – lymphoid hyperplasia, neoplasia, Meckel's diverticulum
Outside the wall	Adhesional – spontaneous, post-inflammatory/infection, postoperative, radiation
	Congenital band
	External mass – neoplastic, inflammatory / abscess
	Hernia
	Superior mesenteric artery syndrome
	Volvulus

Table 34.2 Aetiology of adynamic intestinal obstruction.

Intestinal trauma
abdominal surgery
Extraintestinal trauma
spinal injury
retroperitoneal haematoma
Peritonitis
Ischaemia
Chemical abnormalities
hypokalaemia
diabetic ketoacidosis
renal failure/uraemia

SMALL BOWEL OBSTRUCTION

Clinical presentation

Small bowel obstruction accounts for 4% of surgical emergencies. Common causes include adhesions (60%), hernias (25%) and neoplasms (10%). The majority of patients (70%) with adhesional obstruction settle with conservative management.

History and examination

- History and examination alone can identify the cause in 80% of cases.
- The four cardinal symptoms of obstruction are vomiting, abdominal distension, abdominal pain and absolute constipation.
- Early vomiting suggests high (jejunal) obstruction with late onset vomiting and early constipation occurring in low obstruction.
- Pain is central and colicky (visceral pain) and often settles with prolonged distension due to reduced peristalsis. More severe pain with peritoneal irritation suggests ischaemia or perforation.
- Auscultation reveals high pitched/"tinkling" bowel sounds that may disappear after prolonged obstruction or perforation.

Investigation

- Plasma urea and electrolytes (including creatinine) are essential and arterial blood gas analysis is important to exclude acid-base imbalance.

- Plain abdominal radiographs show distended small bowel with valvulae conniventes and multiple fluid levels in 75% of cases (Figure 34.1). Proximal dilatation and distal collapse help to identify the site of obstruction.
- Contrast studies are useful when the diagnosis is uncertain. Barium provides the best detail but can be harmful in cases of incomplete obstruction or perforation. Water-soluble contrast provides less detail but may have the advantage of promoting peristalsis and relieving adhesional obstruction.

Management

Resuscitation

Early administration of Hartmann's solution or normal saline titred to the amount of extracellular fluid loss (Table 34.3). A urinary catheter facilitates fluid resuscitation.

Nasogastric tube

A nasogastric tube decompresses the gut of fluid and gas.

Indications for surgery

- Uncomplicated obstruction is treated conservatively in 80% providing there are signs of resolution within 24 h.
- Complete small bowel obstruction requires early surgery (<24 h) as delay risks ischaemia, perforation and profound metabolic disturbance.
- Strangulation is common (~40%) in complete obstruction and 10% have no preoperative evidence of ischaemia. If strangulation or perforation is suspected emergency laparotomy following rapid fluid resuscitation is required.

Surgical management

- Surgery should be covered using broad-spectrum antibiotics (cefotaxime 1–2 g tid iv + metronidazole 500 mg tid iv or co-amoxiclav 1 g tid iv).
- Only obstructive adhesions are divided unless otherwise indicated.
- Bowel is decompressed by gentle "milking" of the enteric contents towards a large bore nasogastric tube.
- Areas of necrotic bowel are resected and doubtful viability can be assessed after wrapping the bowel in a moist swab for 30 min (see management of acute mesenteric ischaemia).

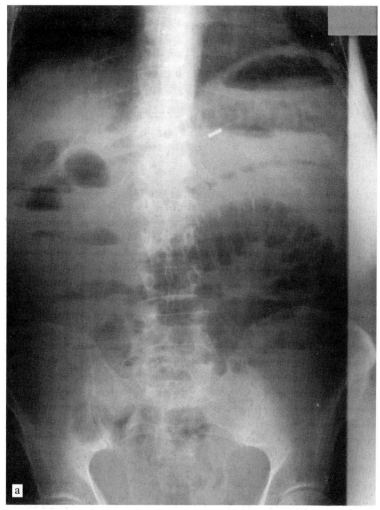

Figure 34.1(a) Erect and supine abdominal *x* ray showing dilated loops of small bowel with multiple fluid levels consistent with small bowel obstruction.

- Malignant or inflammatory strictures (e.g. radiation, Crohn's disease) may not be suitable for resection and require entero-enteral bypass or exteriorisation.
- Methods to reduce recurrent adhesive obstruction include insertion of long enteric tubes and topical application of cellulose-derived polymers.

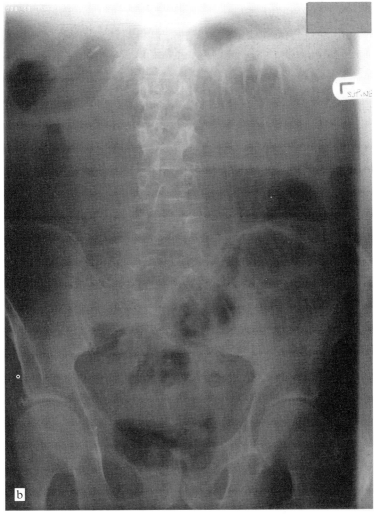

Figure 34.1(b) Supine abdominal *x* ray showing dilated loops of small bowel with multiple fluid levels consistent with small bowel obstruction.

Inoperable obstruction

- In obstruction secondary to advanced abdominal or pelvic malignancy, mortality is high (40%) and surgical decompression is not always achieved or sustained.
- Management includes prolonged nasogastric decompression

Table 34.3 Signs and symptoms of extracellular fluid (ECF) deficit.

ECF deficit	Mild (1–2 l)	Moderate (2–4 l)	Severe (5–9 l)
Symptoms	History of loss	Apathy, anorexia, tachycardia, collapsed veins	Stupor or coma, ileus, pale, hypotensive, cold extremities, absent pulses
Signs	Usually no signs	↓ blood pressure, narrow pulse pressure, ↓ tissue turgor, dry tongue	↓↓ blood pressure, ↓↓ tissue turgor, sunken eyes

Source: Hill GL. Disorders of nutrition and metabolism in clinical surgery, p. 169. (See Further reading) Calculated for normal 70 kg subject. In fat patients the ECF deficit is less. Thin patients have correspondingly higher ECF deficits than normal.

or perhaps preferably continuous administration of analgesia, antiemetics and somatostatin analogues (Octreotide; 200–1200 mg/day).

LARGE BOWEL OBSTRUCTION

Clinical presentation

Commonest causes of colonic obstruction are primary colorectal cancer (53%), volvulus (17%), diverticular disease (12%) and secondary carcinoma (6%). Other causes include ischaemic/inflammatory stricture, hernia, faecal impaction, adhesion and pseudo-obstruction. As obstruction is often closed at both ends (volvulus, competent ileocaecal valve) pressures up to six times higher than in small bowel obstruction can occur thereby increasing the risk of ischaemia and perforation.

History and examination

The symptoms are as for small bowel obstruction with vomiting often presenting as a late feature and constipation or overflow diarrhoea developing early.

Investigation

- Blood analysis.
- Plain abdominal radiography as for small bowel obstruction. Collapsed small bowel, absence of rectal gas and distended colon suggests closed loop obstruction or obstruction with a

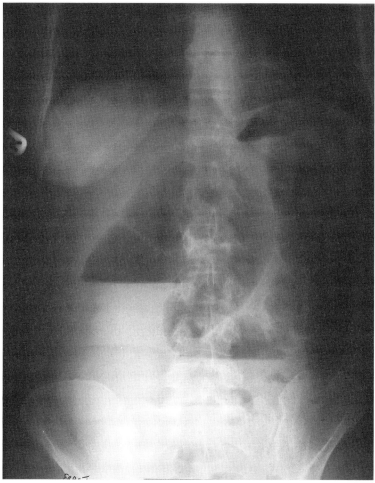

Figure 34.2 An erect plain abdominal *x* ray showing dilated loops of large bowel consistent and fluid levels consistent with large bowel obstruction.

competent ileocaecal valve (Figure 34.2). Sigmoid volvulus presents radiographically as a "bent inner tube" and caecal volvulus as a "coffee bean".

• Proctoscopy/sigmoidoscopy is essential as most lesions are in the distal colon and sigmoid volvuli can usually be decompressed via the rectum.

• Pseudo-obstruction can mimic dynamic obstruction and should be excluded by water-soluble contrast enema or colonoscopy.

- Ultrasonography and CT scanning should be confined to stable patients with a palpable mass in whom additional information influences surgical planning.

Management

Resuscitation

Adequate resuscitation as for small bowel obstruction (see Table 34.3).

Nasogastric tube

Nasogastric intubation may be restricted to those with vomiting and small bowel distension.

Surgery

- Patients with peritoneal irritation require urgent laparotomy.
- Uncomplicated left-sided colonic obstruction due to tumour is best treated by resection (extent dependant on viability) and primary anastomosis. This often requires intraoperative colonic lavage with associated mortality and anastomotic leakage rates of 10% and 5% respectively. Questionable tissue viability and peritoneal contamination favour a Hartmann's procedure.
- Uncomplicated right-sided obstruction is usually treated by right hemicolectomy and primary anastomosis.
- Distal colonic tumours may also be treated temporarily or palliatively by insertion of a self-expanding intraluminal stent, laser ablation or balloon dilatation.

Sigmoid volvulus

- Sigmoid volvulus can be decompressed using the sigmoidoscope in most patients (80–90%) with a flatus tube left in situ for 48 h. A semi-elective resection is indicated if there are further attacks.
- Emergency surgery is associated with higher mortality rates if the bowel is resected and a primary anastomosis performed. A double-barrelled colostomy (Paul-Mickulicz), Hartmann's procedure, non-resectional sigmoid colopexy, or mesosigmoplasty are options in this situation.

Caecal volvulus
- Can also be decompressed endoscopically (colonoscope).
- However, a high incidence of ischaemia and recurrence favours surgery with right hemicolectomy or caecopexy (viable colon) or exteriorisation of both ends (questionable viability).

PSEUDO-OBSTRUCTION (OGILVIE'S SYNDROME)

Clinical Presentation

Pseudo-obstruction is associated with trauma, surgery, cardiovascular compromise (cardiac, cerebrovascular, mesenteric), respiratory disease, metabolic disturbance, intra-abdominal inflammation (e.g. appendicitis, cholecystitis, pancreatitis), neurological disease and the use of certain drugs (e.g. antidepressants, antiparkinsonians, antipsychotics, narcotic analgesia, ganglion blockers). Most cases settle within 6 days with conservative management.

History and Examination
- Typified by obstructive features including abdominal distension (100%), abdominal pain (83%), constipation (51%) and diarrhoea (41%) without any apparent obstructive lesion.
- Usually there is markedly distended abdomen with minimal tenderness.

Investigation
- Associated metabolic and abdominal inflammatory conditions should be excluded.
- Plain abdominal radiographs reveal a markedly distended colon with a 'cut-off' sign most commonly at the splenic flexure.
- Water-soluble contrast enema or colonoscopy may be diagnostic and therapeutic.

Management
Resuscitation
Replace fluid losses and correct metabolic defects (Table 34.2).

Bowel rest

Bowel rest ± total parenteral nutrition can accelerate recovery.

Flatus tube

Insertion of a flatus tube and hyperosmolar enemas can accelerate recovery.

Nasogastric tube

In the absence of vomiting and small bowel distension nasogastric intubation is of little value.

Clinical assessment

Frequent abdominal and radiological assessment is required as increasing and prolonged caecal distension (>12 cm) with abdominal tenderness may herald ischaemia and perforation.

Pharmacotherapy

In cases where recovery is slow neostigmine, cisapride and erythromycin have been shown to promote large bowel peristalsis.

Colonoscopic decompression

Successful in >80% of cases and a further colonoscopy successfully treats the majority of recurrences.

Surgery

If surgical decompression is required a viable colon can be treated by colonoscopic, laparoscopic or open caecostomy. A right hemicolectomy or subtotal colectomy with ileorectal anastomosis may be required for those with ischaemia.

Further reading

1   Bailey I, Tate JJT. Acute conditions of the small bowel and appendix. In: Paterson-Brown S, ed. *A companion to specialist surgical practice: emergency surgery and critical care.* London: WB Saunders, 1997: 187–212.
2   Campbell KL, Munro A. Acute conditions of the large intestine. In: Paterson-Brown S, ed. *A companion to specialist surgical practice: emergency surgery and critical care.* London: WB Saunders, 1997: 151–86.
3   Del Valle Hernandez E. Transanal self-expanding metal stents as an alternative to palliative colostomy in selected patients with malignant obstruction of the left colon. *Br J Surg* 1998; **85**: 232–6.
4   Hill GL. Alimentary tract–obstruction. In: Disorders of nutrition and metabolism in clinical surgery: understanding and management. London: Churchill Livingstone, 1992: 45–70.
5   Lopez-Kostner F, Hool GR, Lavery IC. Management and causes of acute large bowel obstruction. *Surg Clin N Am* 1997; **77**(6): 1265–90.

6 Memon MA, Fitztgibbons RJ. The role of minimal access surgery in the acute abdomen. *Surg Clin N Am* 1997; **77**(6): 1333–53.

7 Ripamonte C. Malignant bowel obstruction in advanced and terminal cancer patients. *Eur J Palliative Care* 1994; **1**: 1–19.

35 Ischaemic bowel

with contributions from John Moorehead, Paul Neilly

Aetiology

The commonest causes of occlusive mesenteric ischaemia include:

- arterial embolus (45%),
- arterial thrombosis (15%) and
- venous thrombosis (5%).

Less common causes include:

- trauma
- surgery
- tumour
- drugs, e.g. digitalis, contraceptives, diuretics, calcium channel blockers, cocaine, vasopressin
- hypercoagulability states,
- endocrine problems, e.g. diabetes, carcinoid
- vasculitis.

In up to 30% of cases the ischaemia is caused by a generalised reduction in splanchnic perfusion secondary to impaired cardiac output (nonocclusive mesenteric ischaemia).

There are two forms of emergency presentation; acute mesenteric ischaemia and ischaemic colitis.

ACUTE MESENTERIC ISCHAEMIA

Natural History

Accounts for 0·1% of acute hospital admissions. Less than 25% have a history of chronic ischaemia (recurrent abdominal pain associated with meals). The high mortality (60% overall; 80% with infarction) is due to delay with the diagnosis and associated co-morbidities (e.g. cardiovascular compromise, arrythmias, systemic atherosclerosis).

History and examination

- Early diagnosis is difficult due to vague symptoms and signs.
- Colicky central abdominal pain with associated vomiting is the main presenting symptom.
- Watery diarrhoea with dark red blood occurs later. In the absence of frank bleeding faecal occult blood testing is usually positive (75%).
- Symptoms are initially more prominent than the physical findings and change with the duration of the ischaemia. Early vague abdominal tenderness progresses to peritonism and ileus with absent bowel sounds when full thickness infarction occurs.
- Initial haemodynamic stability is replaced by features of septi-caemia with metabolic acidosis and eventual multiple organ failure.

Investigation

- Leucocytosis occurs early and biochemistry may show raised concentrations of amylase, lactic dehydrogenase, alkaline phosphatase and creatine kinase. Metabolic acidosis is a feature in advanced cases.
- Plain x rays exclude other causes of pain and can show distended loops of bowel with oedema (thumbprinting). Intramural or portal vein gas represents gangrenous bowel.
- CT scanning is often unhelpful but may show bowel wall oedema and impaired filling of the mesenteric vessels with contrast enhanced studies.
- Special tests include duplex ultrasonography and mesenteric angiography. If the duplex study is positive urgent angiography is required to identify the precise cause of ischaemia and can allow therapeutic manouvres such as vasodilatation, thrombolysis or angioplasty.
- Laparoscopy may be considered in those deemed unsuitable for angiography but normal serosal appearances do not exclude early disease.

Management

A high level of suspicion with prompt resuscitation and investigation is essential.

Resuscitation

- Requires aggressive resuscitation as most patients have moderate/severe fluid deficit with acidosis (see Table 34.2, Chapter 34).
- Early stabilisation of cardiac insufficiency/arrhythmias prior to surgery is important.

Angiography

In nonocclusive mesenteric ischaemia where necrosis is unlikely a conservative regimen using vasodilators infused via angiographically placed catheters may be considered.

Surgery

- Supportive care without bowel resection is most appropriate for elderly patients with infarction of the superior mesenteric artery distribution.
- Others require surgical exploration, resection of gangrenous bowel and restoration of blood flow if possible by embolectomy or thrombectomy. Venous thrombectomy alone rarely gives rewarding results and resection is usually indicated.
- With questionable viability the bowel should be placed in moist swabs at body temperature for 15–30 mins. Viability is determined by the colour of the serosa, visible peristalsis and palpable or Doppler confirmed arterial flow. Alternatively intravenous administration of fluorescein followed by illumination of the bowel using Wood's ultraviolet light can be used. If there is any concern regarding long term viability and integrity of the anastomosis a second look laparotomy/laparoscopy is required after 24–48 h.

ISCHAEMIC COLITIS

Natural History

Usually a transient condition of elderly patients (males>females) but may occur in young patients with low flow states (e.g. hypovolaemia, vasculitis, diabetes, drug abuse). Ischaemia confined to the mucosa and submucosa occurs in 50% with severe transmural necrosis affecting 15%. The commonest site of involvement is the left colon (70%) but recently more frequent ischaemia of the right colon. Mortality is high (50%) and is often related to serious co-morbidity.

History and examination

- Sudden onset of colicky left lower abdominal pain, diarrhoea with dark red rectal bleeding and mucus production is typical.
- Mild localised tenderness, tachycardia and mild pyrexia is common.
- Approximately 15% have features of peritonitis due to gangrenous necrosis, which may progress to circulatory collapse.
- Occasionally these patients pass a large bowel "cast".
- Those with chronic intermittent ischaemia may present with obstruction secondary to stricture formation.

Investigation

- Plain x rays may show thumbprinting in mild/moderate cases. Intramural/portal vein gas occurs with advanced ischaemia.
- Colonoscopy may provide a definitive diagnosis and assessment of severity. In mild disease there is pale mucosa with petechial haemorrhage. Darker/black mucosa with ulceration and sloughing occurs in advanced cases. Colonoscopy increases the risk of perforation and oversufflation may promote ischaemia. Rigid sigmoidoscopy is insufficient, as 75% of ischaemic lesions are proximal to the rectum.
- Angiography and duplex ultrasonography are of little benefit as the major vessels are usually patent.

Management
Conservative treatment
Most cases respond to conservative treatment. This includes:

- bowel rest
- intravenous fluids
- parenteral broad-spectrum antibiotics (cefotaxime 1 – 2 g tid iv + metronidazole 500 mg tid iv or co-amoxiclav 1 g tid iv).

Surgery

- Those with gangrenous colitis or features of increasing abdominal tenderness and toxaemia require laparotomy and radical segmental resection.
- In general the safest policy is to avoid a primary anastomosis.
- The level of resection depends on the extent of mucosal ischaemia as the visual appearance of serosal viability is not sufficient.
- Asymptomatic ischaemic strictures do not require surgical intervention as they rarely cause complete obstruction.
- If surgical treatment of strictures is required resection with primary anastomosis is usually possible.

Further reading

1   Bailey I, Tate JJT. Acute conditions of the small bowel and appendix. In: Paterson-Brown S, ed. *A companion to specialist surgical practice: emergency surgery and critical care.* London: WB Saunders, 1997: 187–212.
2   Campbell KL, Munro A. Acute conditions of the large intestine. In: Paterson-Brown S, ed. *A companion to specialist surgical practic: emergency surgery and critical care.* London: WB Saunders, 1997: 151–86.
3   Memon MA, Fitztgibbons RJ. The role of minimal access surgery in the acute abdomen. *Surg Clin N Am* 1997; 77(6): 1333–53.
4   Schwartz LB, Gewertz BL. Mesenteric ischaemia. *Surg Clin N Am* 1997; 77(2).

36 Inflammatory bowel disease

with contributions from John Moorehead, Paul Neilly

ULCERATIVE COLITIS

Natural history

Patients present with acute attacks (40%) or relapses of bloody diarrhoea (60%). Most then have chronic intermittent disease (65%) with relapses interspersed by symptom-free periods of varying lengths. The requirement for colectomy depends on the extent and duration of disease (total colitis – 36%, left-sided colitis – 38%, distal colitis – 25%, within 5 years of onset – 32%, within 25 years of onset – 65%). Increase in mortality (1·7 times normal population), is dependent on the extent and severity of disease and can be influenced by aggressive medical therapy and early surgical intervention.

History and examination

- Most present with diarrhoea (80%), abdominal pain (70%) or rectal bleeding (60%).
- Weight loss, anaemia and extraintestinal manifestations (arthropathy, iritis, cholangitis, erythema nodosum, pyoderma gangrenosum) are features of chronic severe disease.
- On examination 10% are pyrexic with tenderness localised to the left iliac fossa.
- There may be fresh blood and mucus on digital rectal examination.
- Sigmoidoscopy reveals continuous inflammation often with contact bleeding.
- Severe acute colitis presents as bloody diarrhoea, urgency, tenesmus, abdominal pain, pyrexia and dehydration. There

may be profound hypovolaemia with hyponatraemia, hypokalaemia, hypoalbuminaemia and metabolic acidosis.
- Increasing pain and evidence of peritonism may herald toxic megacolon (5% of severe attacks) or perforation.

Investigation

- Blood analysis includes full blood picture, urea and electrolytes, total protein, albumin, erythrocyte sedimentation rate, C-reactive protein and α_1-acid glycoprotein.
- Blood cultures are required if there is a pyrexia >38°C.
- Faeces should be sent for direct microscopy and culture to exclude infective causes.
- Plain x ray may show oedema with "thumbprinting", submucosal ulceration with "tramlining" and toxic megacolon (transverse colon >5·5 cm).
- Proctoscopy is essential to assess mucosal disease activity and to obtain histological confirmation of the diagnosis.
- Colonoscopy can assess the extent of disease and demonstrate mild inflammatory changes better than radiological studies. Must be used with caution in moderate/severe disease as it can result in worsening of the disease.
- In acute disease a water soluble contrast enema is the investigation of choice to examine the extent and local severity of disease (Figure 36.1).

Assessment of severity

Severity of symptoms generally correlates with severity and extent of disease. The most commonly used scoring system is that devised by Truelove and Witts:

Severe   ≥6 motions/day (with blood)
            systemic disease (fever >37·5°C, pulse >90/min, anaemia <9 g/dl)
            ESR > 30 mm/h
Moderate ≥4–6 motions/day (with or without blood)
            minimal systemic disease
Mild   <4 motions/day (with or without blood)
            no systemic disease
            ESR normal

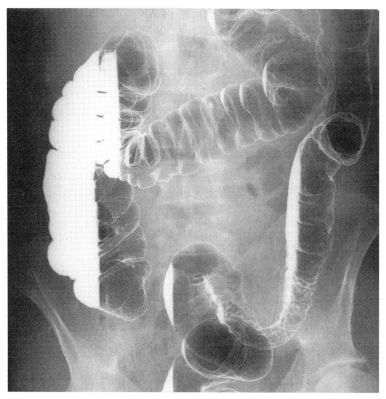

Figure 36.1 Barium enema showing ulceration and pseudopolyp formation from mid-transverse colon to rectum consistent with ulcerative colitis.

Management

Medical therapy

Mild attack

- Outpatient treatment.
- Topical steroid or 5-aminosalicylic acid (5-ASA) enemas.
- Oral 5-ASA preparations (1·5–2 g/day) are indicated for extensive disease.
- Relapses in those already using a 5-ASA preparation are treated with oral steroids (prednisolone 20 mg/day) and reduced by 5 mg each week after 2 weeks of treatment.

Moderate attack

- Usually responds to oral steroids (prednisolone 40–60mg/day) and reduced by 5 mg each week after 2 weeks of treatment.

- Topical steroid or 5-aminosalicylic acid (5-ASA) enemas.
- Oral 5-ASA preparations (1·5–2 g/day) are indicated for extensive disease.
- Some patients with systemic involvement will require hospitalisation.

Severe attack

- Requires hospitalisation.
- Intravenous steroids (hydrocortisone 100 mg/6 h, methylprednisolone 16 mg/6 h).
- Topical steroid enemas.
- Improvement should occur within 5–7 days and oral prednisolone then started (40–60 mg / day).
- Those failing to respond should be considered for intravenous cyclosporin 4 mg/kg/day and if successful continued orally for 3 months (6 mg/kg/day).
- Oral nutrition does not prevent resolution but may induce discomfort. Oral elemental/semi-elemental diets or total parenteral nutrition may be indicated during the acute phase.
- Antibiotics (cefotaxime 1–2 g tid iv + metronidazole 500 mg tid iv or co-amoxiclav 1 g tid iv) are only required if the blood culture is positive or a complication occurs (toxic megacolon/perforation) Please see below.
- Steroid dependent disease or those with multiple relapses may benefit from azathioprine (efficacy in 70%; onset of action about 6–12 weeks; dose 2–2·5 mg/kg/day).

Indications for surgery

Approximately 25% of patients with acute disease require a colectomy. Indications for emergency surgery include:

- failure to respond to maximal steroid or cyclosporin therapy,
- toxic megacolon not settling within 24 h of maximal medical therapy (50%),
- perforation,
- massive haemorrhage.

Surgical options

The three main surgical options in ulcerative colitis are:

- subtotal colectomy/panproctocolectomy with ileostomy formation,
- abdominal colectomy with ileorectal anastomosis,
- panproctocolectomy with ileal pouch-anal anastomosis.

In acute severe disease subtotal colectomy and ileostomy formation is the preferred option.

COMPLICATIONS OF ULCERATIVE COLITIS

Toxic megacolon

Clinical presentation

- Criteria for diagnosis of toxic megacolon are:
  - radiological evidence of colonic distension > 6 cm in diameter (Figure 36.2)

  plus at least three of the four following conditions:
  - fever higher than 38·6°C
  - heart rate > 120 bpm
  - neutrophil leucocytosis > 10 500 cells/mm
  - anaemia.

  plus at least one sign of toxicity:
  - dehydration
  - mental changes
  - electrolyte disturbance
  - hypotension.
- On examination, patients may have pyrexia, postural hypotension, tenderness over the distribution of the colon, rebound tenderness, abdominal distension, bowels sounds sluggish or absent.

Management

- Nil by mouth.
- Nasogastric tube suction.
- Intravenous fluids to correct metabolic disorders, usually hypokalaemia, hyponatraemia, hypochlorhydria and hypovolaemia.
- Cefotaxime 1–2 g tid iv + metronidazole 500 mg tid iv.
- Most clinicians would continue steroids (hydrocortisone 100 mg/6 h, methylprednisolone 16 mg/6 h).
- If medical therapy is successful during the first 24–48 h, an improvement in the signs of clinical toxicity and a decrease in the diameter of the dilated colon should be seen.
- If there is no improvement, then surgery is indicated. The most usual procedure is colonic resection and an ileostomy.

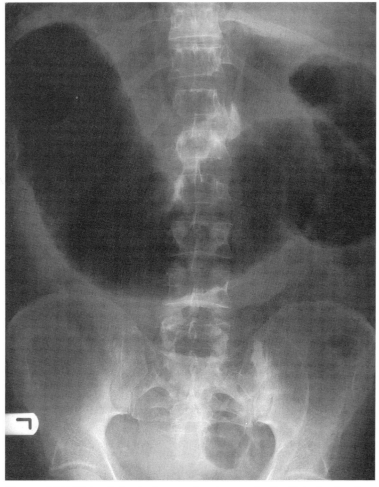

Figure 36.2 Plain abdominal x ray showing markedly dilated colon in a patient with ulcerative colitis consistent with toxic megacolon.

Perforation

- Commonly complicates toxic megacolon but can occur in severe ulcerative colitis without toxic megacolon.
- Mortality is about 40%.
- Clinical features include increasing pain, signs of peritonitis, loss of hepatic dullness on percussion, clinical deterioration with pyrexia, tachycardia, hypotension, air under the diaphragm on abdominal x ray.

- Administer antibiotics: cefotaxime 1–2 g tid iv + metronidazole 500 mg tid iv
- Most patients should undergo surgery (see Surgical options above).

Stricture

- Clinically important strictures are relatively uncommon in ulcerative colitis.
- They tend to occur in patients with extensive disease and continuous symptoms without remission.
- Symptoms include an increase in diarrhoea and faecal incontinence.
- Patients should undergo a colonoscopy and biopsy.
- If malignancy is suspected or confirmed, they should undergo resection.

CROHN'S DISEASE

Natural history

Crohn's disease involves the small bowel only in 30%, colon only in 25% and both small and large bowel in 45%. In approximately 65% the terminal ileum is affected. Usually there is a long history of diarrhoea and abdominal pain but approximately 10% of patients present with acute disease. One third present with complications (abscess – 15%; fistula – 15%; obstruction – 3%). Small bowel and colonic Crohn's disease are both progressive but colonic disease has fewer complications and more extraintestinal manifestations. Megacolon occurs in about 10% of patients with Crohn's colitis.

Mortality is increased (twice that of normal population) and is due to complications such as malnutrition, malignant change, amyloidosis and postoperative complications. The differences between ulcerative colitis and Crohn's disease are shown in Table 36.1.

History and examination

- The commonest symptoms on acute presentation are abdominal pain (95%), diarrhoea (90%), weight loss (85%) and fever (56%).

Table 36.1 Differences between ulcerative and Crohn's disease

Assessment	Ulcerative colitis	Crohn's disease
Clinical features	Rectal bleeding in 60% Anal lesions in 25% Perianal fistulae uncommon Pain & tenderness right iliac fossa Weight loss in 20%	Rectal bleeding in 40% (colitis 60%) Anal lesions in 40% (colonic 75%) Perianal fistulae in 5-10% Pain & tenderness left iliac fossa Weight loss in 70%
Radiology	Inflammatory polyps Continuous change Fibrous strictures rare	Rarely inflammatory polyps Segmental change (80%) Fibrous strictures common

Endoscopy	Continuous inflammation
	 Rectum involved in 100%
	 Terminal ileum involved in 10%
	 Mucosa –
	    vascular
	    granular & ulcerated
	    no fissures
		Patchy inflammation
		 Rectum involved in 20%
		 Terminal ileum involved in 65%
		 Mucosa –
		    not vascular
		    discrete ulcers
		    cobblestones & fissures

Pathology	Mucosal ulcers Crypt abscesses common Mucosal/submucosal involvement Fibrous strictures rare No granulomata	Deep fissures Crypt abscesses rare Transmural involvement Fibrous strictures common Granulomas in 60%

- Abdominal pain is often postprandial and is usually central (colicky) or localised to the area of maximal inflammation, e.g. right iliac fossa (dull ache).
- Rectal bleeding is more common in Crohn's colitis whereas proximal small bowel disease often presents with vomiting.
- Examination reveals maximal tenderness at the site of inflammation and an inflammatory mass may be palpable (usually right iliac fossa).

Investigation

- Broad based blood and faecal analysis is required including assessment of the acute phase inflammatory markers (see investigation of ulcerative colitis).
- Plain x rays may show segmental oedema, obstruction or toxic dilatation.
- Small bowel disease is best examined by small bowel enema (enteroclysis) (Figure 36.3).
- Advantages of colonoscopy include histological differentiation

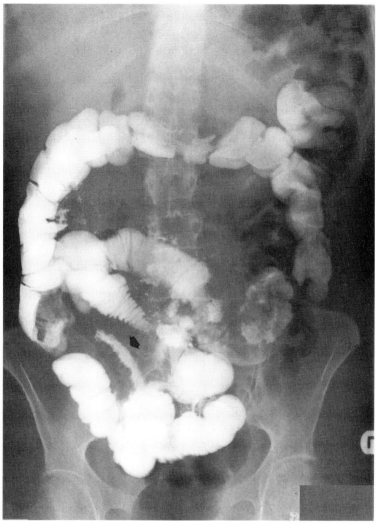

Figure 36.3 Small bowel series showing stricturing, rosethorn ulceration and displacement of adjacent loops of bowel in terminal ileum (arrow) consistent with Crohn's disease.

between ulcerative colitis and Crohn's colitis and assessment of the terminal ileum.

- Ultrasonography and CT scanning are useful to assess inflammatory masses by excluding abscess formation and defining the response to medical therapy.

211

Assessment of severity

Features most related to severity in order are pulse rate, temperature, systemic complications, abdominal pain, abdominal distension and bowel habit. The most useful severity scoring system is the Harvey-Bradshaw Index which assesses:

General well-being   0–3 (0 good, 3 bad)
Abdominal pain   0–4
Loose motions/24 h   0 +
Abdominal mass   0–3 (none, ill defined, easily palpable, tender)
Complications   0–8 (abscess, anal fissure, apthous ulcers, arthralgia, erythema nodosum, fistula, pyoderma gangrenosum, uveitis)

Useful serum markers include ESR, albumin, C reactive protein and α_1-acid glycoprotein. Haemoglobin and platelet counts are also markers of disease activity.

Management

Medical therapy

The treatment is similar to that for ulcerative colitis.

- In addition oral metronidazole (400 mg tid) is useful for colonic and perianal Crohn's disease.
- Severe disease usually warrants admission to hospital for bowel rest (in small bowel disease) and intravenous steroids (hydrocortisone 100 mg/6 h, methylprednisolone 16 mg/6 h). Providing there is an adequate response after 1 week oral prednisolone is started (40–60 mg/day) with a reducing regimen as for ulcerative colitis.
- With steroid dependant disease budesonide (9 mg od) or azathioprine (2–2·5 mg/kg/day) may prevent relapse.
- Oral 5-ASA medication is less effective in Crohn's disease but should also be started as early as possible at 1·5–2 g/day.
- Cyclosporin (4 mg/kg/day intravenously, 6–8 mg/kg/day orally) should be considered for complicated perianal sepsis and if successful must be withdrawn slowly (6–12 months). Efficacy is much less convincing than for ulcerative colitis.
- In contrast to ulcerative colitis there is good evidence that nutritional therapy, and in particular enteral formulations (elemental, semi-elemental and polymeric), are equivalent to steroid therapy in reducing disease activity. They can therefore be used as an adjunct to standard medical therapy.

Surgical therapy

- Surgery is restricted to patients with failed medical treatment and complications (persistent obstruction, free-perforation and haemorrhage). Surgery is required for ~75% of those with Crohn's disease and individuals may expect on average one operation per decade of disease.
- The principles of surgery are as follows:
  1 Preserve as much bowel as possible (stricturoplasty and avoidance of resection).
  2 Early surgical intervention reduces mortality and morbidity.
  3 Large anastomoses reduce local recurrence.
  4 Allow spontaneous or postoperative enterocutaneous fistulae to mature.
  5 In malnourished patients with sepsis (perforation/abscesses/fistulae) exteriorise rather than anastomose.

COMPLICATIONS OF CROHN'S DISEASE

Abscesses

Clinical presentation

- The typical presentation is fever and abdominal pain. The location and quality of the pain is determined by the location of the abscess.
- Physical findings include tenderness and abdominal mass.
- Diagnosis is usually made by CT scan.

Management

- Administer antibiotics: cefotaxime 1–2 g tid iv + metronidazole 500 mg tid iv.
- The abscess can be initially drained percutaneously under CT or ultrasound scan guidance.
- Surgical therapy is required for definitive treatment. The portion of involved intestine is resected.

Fistulas

Clinical presentation

- Most fistulas are enteroenteric or enterocutaneous with smaller numbers that are enterovesical or enterovaginal.
- Most enteroenteric fistulas seldom cause significant symptoms but those of large diameter may cause malabsorption, diarrhoea and weight loss.

- Pain and diarrhoea in patients with enteroenteric fistulas are usually caused by active Crohn's inflammation and not by the mere presence of the fistula.
- Rectovaginal fistulas cause a foul vaginal discharge. Larger fistulas result in the passage of gas and stool through the vagina. They can be identified by proctoscopy, speculum examination or barium enema.
- Enterovesicular fistulas may result in gas in the urine and recurrent urinary tract infections. Diagnosis may be made by barium enema, small bowel series, cystoscopy or intravenous pyelogram.

Management

- Asymptomatic fistulas require no treatment.
- Total parenteral nutrition (TPN) may induce fistula closure but often recur after the TPN is stopped.
- Immunosuppression with azathioprine can close fistulas but often recur when the drug is stopped.
- Infliximab (a TNF – α antagonist) is effective in closing fistulas.
- Surgery includes resection of the segment involved with active disease.
- Rectovaginal fistula – metronidazole leads to healing in some. Definitive therapy usually requires surgery – diverting colostomy or abdominal perineal resection.
- Enterovesicular fistulas – definitive surgery, resection of the involved segment of bowel, is recommended.

Obstruction

Clinical presentation

- Presents with cramping abdominal pain and diarrhoea that worsen after meals and resolve with fasting. Symptoms start off as intermittent episodes followed by more severe episodes accompanied by nausea and vomiting.
- Strictures may be evaluated by small bowel series, barium enema or colonoscopy.

Management

- For acute obstruction, see Chapter 34.
- Steroids may help if acute inflammation is an important component but does not help if the stricture is fibrotic.

- If the obstruction does not settle with nasogastric suction and steroids, dilation or surgery is necessary.
- Endoscopic balloon dilatation can be attempted if the stricture is short and accessible.
- Surgery includes either resection or stricturoplasty.

Perianal disease

Clinical presentation

- Fistulas present with drainage of serous or mucous material.
- Perianal abscesses present with pain that is exacerbated by defaecation, sitting, or walking. There is redness and pain in the perianal region with tenderness on digital examination.
- Adequate assessment of perianal disease usually requires proctoscopic examination under anaesthesia.
- Barium enema may reveal the course of fistulas.
- CT scans are useful in defining the presence and extent of perianal abscesses.

Management

- Sitz baths.
- External drainage with setons or drains.
- Minimise disease activity of Crohn's with medical management (see above).
- Metronidazole (250 mg qid) is very effective in healing perianal disease. Discontinuation results in recurrence in the majority of patients.
- Other surgical approaches should be considered if the above fails: partial anal sphincterotomy, marsupialise all the fistulous tracts, faecal diversion by colostomy.

References

1   Bailey I, Tate JJT. Acute conditions of the small bowel and appendix. In: Paterson-Brown S, ed. *A companion to specialist surgical practice: emergency surgery and critical care*. London: WB Saunders, 1997: 187–212.
2   Campbell KL, Munro A. Acute conditions of the large intestine. In: Paterson-Brown S, ed. *A companion to specialist surgical practice: emergency surgery and critical care*. London: WB Saunders, 1997: 151–86.
3   Forbes A (ed). *Clinicians' Guide to Inflammatory Bowel Disease*. London: Chapman & Hall, 1997.
4   Memon MA, Fitztgibbons RJ. The role of minimal access surgery in the acute abdomen. *Surg Clin N Am* 1997; 77(6): 1333–53.

37 Infectious diarrhoea

with contributions from John Moorehead, Paul Neilly

Natural history

Infection is the most common cause of diarrhoea and is most problematic in children and the elderly. Complications include dehydration, malnutrition, metabolic deficit, haemorrhage (dysentery), toxic megacolon, perforation and disseminated/metastatic infection. Infectious diarrhoea can be distinguished from inflammatory bowel disease by demonstration of the pathogen. The pathogens can be subdivided into bacteria, viruses and parasites. This section concentrates on the common virulent pathogens.

History

- Relevant history includes foreign travel, contact with carriers (humans, cattle, sheep, pigs, birds and dogs), contaminated food (unpasteurised/unsterilised dairy produce, uncooked meat, seafood and vegetables, unwashed and unpeeled fruit), antibiotic therapy (pseudomembranous colitis) and male homosexuality ("gay bowel").
- Colicky abdominal pain, watery/bloody diarrhoea, excess mucus, tenesmus, pyrexia are common symptoms. Nausea, vomiting, muscle pains and headaches may accompany the diarrhoeal illness and commonly precede it in viral gastroenteritis.
- Bacterial and viral illnesses usually resolve within 5 days whereas symptoms from parasitic infection are more insidious.

Investigation

- Mild self-limiting illness requires no formal investigation unless other inflammatory or malignant conditions are suspected.
- In prolonged (>2 weeks) or severe illness the faeces are examined by direct microscopy looking for erythrocytes and polymorphonuclear cells (evidence of invasive pathogens), ova and parasites. In the absence of visible pathogens the faeces should be cultured.
- DNA probes and PCR may be required to identify specific pathogens (Table 37.1).
- Proctoscopy with biopsy should be performed to exclude idiopathic inflammatory bowel disease.
- Common small bowel pathogens include *Escherichia coli* (enterotoxigenic and enteropathogenic), *vibrio cholerae*, rotavirus, Norwalk virus and *Giardia*. Colonic pathogens include *Shigella*, *Escherichia coli* (enteroinvasive and enterohaemorrhagic), and *Entamoeba histolytica* and *Clostridium dificile*.

Management

General measures and hydration

- Most patients settle with supportive therapy.
- Encourage food intake (avoiding dairy products and caffeine) with oral rehydration therapy to replace fluid and electrolyte losses including bicarbonate and potassium deficits (Table 37.1).
- Oral solutions include WHO oral rehydration salts (British National Formulary), Dioralyte (Rhône-Poulenc Rorer, Kent) and Rehidrat (Searle, Buckinghamshire).
- Intravenous therapy is reserved for the severely dehydrated and those unable to tolerate oral rehydration.

Antimotility drugs

Antimotility drugs (loperamidc, codeine, co-phenotrope) should be considered in mild/moderate disease and of these loperamide has the least side effects.

Antibiotics

Antibiotics are only required for severely ill individuals with systemic manifestations of disease. They may also be considered for severe dysentery, prolonged disease (>2 weeks) and virulent

Table 37.1 Specific features and therapy for common infective diarrhoeal illnesses.

Agent	Species	Specific features	Specific treatment
Bacteria	Escherichia coli	Usually affects small bowel. Symptoms depend on serotype. Often presents as traveller's diarrhoea. Invasive and haemorrhagic forms may present like shigella dysentery	Ciprofloxacin 500 mg; single dose or b.d. × 3 days or co-trimoxazole 960 mg b.d. × 3 days
	Campylobacter jejuni	Mild diarrhoea to severe dysentery. May be persistent in HIV patients. Diagnosis by stool culture	Ciprofloxacin 500 mg b.d. or erythromycin 250–500 mg q.i.d. × 5–7 days
	Salmonella spp.	May present as: gastroenteritis, bacteraemia, disseminated disease, Typhoid fever, asymptomatic carrier. Early diagnosis by blood culture. Later by faecal culture	Ciprofloxacin 500 mg or co-trimoxazole 960 mg b.d. × 5 days. For typhoid fever use. Chloramphenicol 500 mg q.i.d. × 10–14 days
	Shigella spp.	Small bowel phase – watery diarrhoea × 3–5 days Colonic phase – dysentery and tenesmus +/− toxic megacolon. Diagnosis by stool culture or ELISA for toxin	If resistant to ampicillin 500 mg q.i.d. and co-trimoxazole 960 mg b.d. use ciprofloxacin 500 mg b.d. × 5 days
	Vibrio cholerae	Usually mild disease but can give sudden onset severe "rice water" diarrhoea. Diagnosed by direct microscopy, antisera immobilisation and faecal culture	Tetracycline 250 mg q.i.d. × 3–5 days or doxycycline 200–300 mg single dose
	Yersinia enterocolitica	May give prolonged diarrhoea with x ray features of terminal ileitis thus confusing with IBD. Diagnosis by culture of faeces, blood or mesenteric nodes (if surgery for appendicitis)	Ciprofloxicin 500 mg b.d. or co-trimoxazole 960 mg b.d. × 3-5 days
	Clostridium dificile	Secondary to antibiotic therapy. Presents as pseudomembranous colitis. Diagnosis by culture, enzyme immunoassay	Withdraw causative antibiotic. Metronidazole 400 mg t.i.d. or vancomycin 125 mg q.i.d. × 6 days

		Clinical features / Diagnosis	Treatment
Viruses	Rotavirus	Mainly children. Usually starts with vomiting. Watery diarrhoea. Diagnosis by immunoassay, PCR or nucleic acid probes	Supportive care/rehydration
	Norwalk virus	Usually mild illness. No routine diagnostic test	Supportive care/rehydration
Parasites	*Entamoeba histolytica*	Colonises colonic wall causing ulceration and dysentery. May invade liver. Diagnosis by repeated faecal analysis	Metronidazole 800 mg t.i.d. × 10 days followed by diloxanide furoate 500 mg t.i.d. × 10 days.
	Giardia duodenalis	Upper abdominal pain preceding diarrhoea/dysentery. Diagnosis by direct microscopy of faeces or jejunal biopsy	Metronidazole 400 mg t.i.d. × 5 days or tinidazole 2 g single dose
	Roundworms	May enter via skin or gut. Invades lung. Abdominal pain with peritonitis due migration from gut. Diagnosis by faecal analysis	Treatment specific to worm type or mebendazole 100 mg b.d. × 3 days
	Tapeworms	Infection by oral intake. Diagnosis by faecal analysis	Praziquantel 20 mg/kg/niclosamide 2 g single dose
	Schistosomiasis	Infection by skin penetration. Intestinal features occur late. Acute and chronic dysentery with ulceration and polyps. Diagnosis by repeated faecal analysis.	Praziquantel 40-60mg/kg in 2 or 3 divided doses depending on fluke type

pathogens. Specific features of infective diarrhoea and therapies are outlined in Table 37.1 and in the section on specific causes below.

SPECIFIC THERAPY OF INFECTIVE DIARRHOEAS

Cholera

Clinical presentation

Cholera is usually considered to be a disease of the tropics, particularly Asia and parts of Africa. Outbreaks have been recorded in Southern Europe and the disease may be introduced into the UK by travellers.

The diagnosis is usually confirmed by the finding of motile organisms of Vibrio cholerae in freshly passed stool specimens.

Management

- Appropriate and prompt oral rehydration is the mainstay of therapy WHO/UNICEF solution (see Chapter 7, Table 7.3) should be given in a dose of 50 ml/kg body weight over the first 4 h followed by 100 ml/kg daily until diarrhoea stops and the infection has cleared.
- Intravenous reydration is indicated in the presence of circulatory collapse when 3–5 l of Ringer's lactate solution or the WHO-approved "diarrhoea treatment solution" consisting of NaCl 4.0 g, KCl 1.0 g and glucose 9.0 g/l should be administered until oral fluids can be tolerated.
- In some cases, tetracycline 250 mg qds for 3–5 days or doxycycline 200–300 mg single dose can accelerate clearance of the infection but growing resistance is a problem.

Escherichia coli

Clinical presentation

Escherichia coli is responsible for enteric disease and acute diarrhoeal outbreaks are of four main types:

- *Enterotoxigenic E. coli (ETEC)* produces diarrhoea associated with massive secretion of water and electrolytes into the intestinal lumen. The clinical syndromes are:
  - a cholera-like ilness,
  - "traveller's diarrhoea" and

– children's diarrhoeal illnesses.

- *Enteroinvasive E. coli* cause a shigella – like illness (see below)
- *Enteropathogenic E. coli (EPEC)* usually affects children under 2 years old and causes outbreaks in nurseries.
- *Enterohaemorrhagic E. coli* produces a cytotoxin similar to shigella. It is usually linked with contaminated food.

Management

- Oral and sometimes intravenous fluid replacement is required in severe cases.
- If systemic infection is present oral ampicillin 2 g daily or co-trimoxazole 960 mg twice daily or ciprofloxacin 500 mg single dose or bd should be given for 3 days.
- Severe sepsis can occur and requires iv gentamicin 2–5 mg/kg or tobramycin 3–5 mg/kg 8 h.

Salmonella
Clinical presentation
Salmonella causes
- Typhoid and paratyphoid fever
- Enterocolitis (which may mimic ulcerative colitis)
- Septicaemia
- Food poisoning
- A carrier state.

Management
- Most cases are self limiting and require symptomatic and supportive therapy only.
- In cases of *S. typhi* (typhoid fever), chloramphenicol 75 mg/kg body weight is the drug of choice.
- Oral antibiotics are not indicated in cases of salmonella food poisoning.

Shigellosis
Clinical presentation
Shigellosis or bacillary dysentery is caused by Gram negative bacilli from the species Shigella. The infection is associated with a short incubation period of 2–3 days. The diarrhoeal illness is acute, associated with crampy abdominal pain and passage of bloody stools. Sigmoidoscopy shows a hyperaemic bowel mucosa with

ulcers again mimicking an acute case of non-specific inflammatory bowel disease.

Management
- Treatment is supportive.
- In severe cases, ampicillin 50–100 mg/kg in children and 2 g daily in adults can be given.
- Alternative antibiotics include cotrimoxazole or ciprofloxacin (see Table 37.1).

Pseudomembranous colitis
Clinical presentation
Pseudomembranous colitis usually results from the use of any antibiotic particularly lincomycin, ampicillin and cephalosporins. Diarrhoea is usually severe and watery. The diagnosi is established by finding Clostridium difficile toxin in fresh stool samples.

Management
- The treatment is or metronidazole 400 mg tds or vancomycin 125–500 mg qds for 1 or 2 weeks.
- Both antibiotics are very effective with response rates of over 90%. Metronidazole is the drug of first choice as it is cheaper and vancomycin can be used in cases that do not respond to metronidazole.

Further reading
1 Farthing MJG. Gut infections. In: Pounder RE, ed. *Recent advances in gastroenterology.* Edinburgh: Churchill Livingstone, 1994: 1–21.

38 Diverticular disease

with contributions from John Moorehead, Paul Neilly

Introduction

Diverticulae develop due to raised intracolonic pressure caused by low fibre diets and slow colonic transit. Each diverticulum is a hernia of mucosa through a region of weakness in the muscularis propria (e.g. entry points of vessels). Most are left-sided (sigmoid colon) with right-sided involvement more common in the Far East. The incidence increases with age and affects 33% of patients over 60 years but the majority are asymptomatic. Uncomplicated disease usually presents with lower abdominal pain and altered bowel function. Acute presentations are related to complications including diverticulitis, perforation (free or concealed), fistula, bleeding and bowel obstruction.

DIVERTICULITIS

Natural history

Acute diverticulitis accounts for 1% of emergency hospital admissions. Of these 50% have had no previous symptoms and only 7% required a previous hospital admission. With conservative management 80% settle and almost 45% remain free of symptoms after a single attack. However 32% of patients develop severe complications within 5 years of presentation with almost 8% dying from recurrent diverticulitis.

History and examination

- Visceral colicky pain progresses to sharp parietal pain with tenderness localised to the area of maximal inflammation (left iliac fossa in sigmoid disease). Pain is often eased with defaecation and >60% have altered bowel function.

- Left-sided tenderness is common on rectal examination and most are pyrexic with a mild leucocytosis.

Investigations

- Useful emergency studies include full blood cell count, plain x rays (erect chest and supine abdomen) and urinalysis with direct microscopy. Urinary tract infection suggests a colovesical fistula.
- Water soluble contrast enema may confirm the diagnosis and identify complications (e.g. perforation or fistula). Barium studies give better definition but may increase the morbidity associated with perforation and emergency surgery.
- Double contrast barium studies or colonoscopy (>2 weeks after the acute phase) can define the extent and severity of disease and exclude malignant lesions.
- Ultrasonography and computed tomography provide a method by which pericolic masses can be examined and diverticular abscesses drained.

Management

General measures

Mild cases may be treated at home but severe pain, significant alteration in bowel habit and evidence of complications justifies admission to hospital.

Supportive therapy

This includes analgesia and intravenous fluids. Nasogastric tubes are only required for profuse vomiting or obstruction.

Antibiotics

Treatment should be directed against aerobes and anaerobes. Appropriate antibiotics if there are peritoneal signs include: cefotaxime 1–2 g tid iv + metronidazole 500 mg tid iv or co-amoxiclav 1 g tid iv. Therapy should be maintained for 5–7 days. If there are no peritoneal signs, appropriate antibiotics are: oral co-amoxiclav 1 g tid, or ciprofloxacin 500 mg bid for 5–7 days.

Surgery

In the acute phase surgery is reserved for those failing to respond to maximal medical therapy or with features of generalised or faecal peritonitis (see management of perforation).

PERFORATION

Natural history

Over 20% admitted to hospital with diverticular disease have peritonitis due to a perforation. There is a high mortality rate (33%) which rises to over 50% in those with faecal peritonitis (one third of all peritonitis cases). Of those offered surgery there is a 30% postoperative mortality.

History and examination

- Perforation precedes abscess formation but rupture of the abscess wall (purulent peritonitis) or free intraperitoneal rupture of a diverticulum (faecal peritonitis) presents with severe acute abdominal pain, dehydration, fever, tachycardia, generalised tenderness with guarding and absent bowel sounds.
- Severe hypovolaemia and septicaemia with either leucocytosis or leucopenia and acidosis are classical features of faecal peritonitis.
- Patients with purulent peritonitis are generally less unwell.

Investigation

- In those with fulminant septicaemia or severe generalised peritonitis further investigations should not prevent early surgical intervention.
- Serum urea and electrolyte determination and arterial blood gas analysis may influence medical management.
- Perforation may be confirmed on plain x ray or following extravasation of contrast during enema studies.

Management
Antibiotics

- With evidence of perforation but abdominal signs limited to a single quadrant supportive therapy with antibiotic treatment is appropriate (as for uncomplicated diverticulitis).
- Widespread peritonitis or septicaemia requires triple therapy including ampicillin, metronidazole and an aminoglycoside such as gentamicin.

Resuscitation

Vigorous fluid resuscitation to maintain a urinary output of >60 ml/h with compensation for hyperventilation and pyrexia (500–1000 ml extra/24 h).

Surgery

- Laparoscopy can assist with the diagnosis, assess disease severity, examine for evidence of perforation and provide a means of peritoneal toilet.
- Definitive treatment for purulent and faecal peritonitis is surgical whether by laparoscopically assisted surgery or by conventional laparotomy.
- Recently there has been a move away from three stage procedures involving drainage and proximal stoma formation at the initial emergency operation. There is improved control of sepsis and increased survival with primary colonic resection.
- Laparoscopic assisted colonic resection may reduce morbidity and the length of postoperative hospitalisation.

ABSCESS

Natural history

Most if not all abscesses represent contained perforations of diverticulae. They complicate acute diverticulitis in 11% of cases most of which develop within the mesocolon. The mortality is 12% in this group.

History and examination

- Pain is localised to the visceral and parietal innervation of the abscess wall. Typical features of abscesses occur (swinging

fevers, rigors, weight loss) with additional symptoms of dysuria, urinary frequency, tenesmus, and dyspareunia in those with pelvic collections. Pus may be discharged from rectum, vagina or urethra.
- These abscesses may be palpable by rectal or vaginal examination. Above the pelvic brim they may present as tender masses causing oedema and erythema of the skin.
- Compression or inflammatory infiltration of small bowel can lead to mechanical obstruction or ileus.

Investigation
- CT scanning and ultrasonography can differentiate an abscess from a diverticular phlegmon. Enhanced CT examination using water-soluble contrast enema may identify the site of perforation.

Management
Conservative treatment
This requires complete bowel rest, intravenous fluids and antibiotics as recommended for simple diverticulitis. Small pericolic abscesses may require no further treatment.

Surgery
Larger lesions and those failing to respond to conservative management require open or percutaneous drainage. Recently there has been a move towards radiological percutaneous drainage with elective resection and primary anastomosis when the acute phase has settled.

FISTULA

Natural history
Diverticulitis is the most common cause of a fistula arising from the colon and the most common destination is the bladder (colovesical fistula). Other types of fistula include colocutaneous (abdominal wall, buttock, groin or perineum), colovaginal, coloenteric, coloureteral, colouterine, colosalpingeal. Fistulation is the main feature in 10% of those with acute diverticulitis and may complicate drainage of a diverticular abscess.

227

History and examination

- There is often a history of abdominal pain and fever suggestive of a preceding abscess.
- The symptoms attributed to the fistula are related to the viscus with which the colon communicates. For example colovesical fistulas present with repeated urinary infections (75%), pneumaturia (60%) and occasionally faecaluria.
- Many present acutely with diverticulitis and the fistula is identified unexpectedly at laparotomy.

Investigations

- Contrast enemas will only show a fistula track in 50%. Analysis of the urine for barium deposits following the barium enema may confirm the diagnosis.
- Colocutaneous fistula may be further assessed by fistulography.
- CT scanning may assess disease severity and identify fistulae (air in bladder).
- Cystoscopy may show an abnormality in up to 90% but is rather non-specific demonstrating the opening in less than 50%.
- Colonoscopy excludes other causes of fistula (e.g. malignancy, Crohn's disease).

Management

Surgery

- Most fistulas do not require emergency surgery and deferral allows the acute inflammatory process to resolve.
- The priority in fistula surgery is to excise the origin of disease after pinching it off the secondary organ. This is then oversewn and/or drained (e.g. by urinary catheter $+/-$ pelvic drain in colovesical fistula).
- In emergency cases if the sepsis is contained and colonic irrigation is feasible the colon should be resected with a primary anastomosis.

HAEMORRHAGE

(See Chapter 6)

Natural history

Although previously considered a rare feature of diverticular disease the accepted overall incidence is about 15%. Diverticular disease however is the commonest cause of severe colonic haemorrhage. Most are otherwise asymptomatic elderly individuals with no previous known diverticular disease but often a history of hypertension, ischaemic heart disease, diabetes and oral anticoagulant usage. Patients rarely have chronic intermittent bleeding and anaemia. Most have bleeding which stops spontaneously; 25% will rebleed but it is rarely a cause of death.

History and examination

Usually present with painless rectal bleeding and evidence of mild hypovolaemia. Most are haemodynamically stable (84%).

Investigations

- Full blood picture and coagulation status should be determined.
- Proctoscopy/rigid sigmoidoscopy will help exclude bleeding rectal causes such as haemorrhoids or inflammatory bowel disease.
- Further investigations should follow the previously discussed pattern in Chapter 6.

Management

Conservative treatment

- Most of these patients are elderly with associated co-morbidity and will therefore only be suitable for conservative management.
- If the patient is stable and estimated blood loss less than 3 1 conservative management should continue.
- Persistent bleeding may also respond to colonoscopy with diathermy coagulation.
- See Section I for recommended resuscitative measures.

Surgery

- Unless otherwise contraindicated unstable patients with prompt persistent bleeding require surgery.
- If the site of haemorrhage cannot be identified an abdominal

colectomy with ileorectal anastomosis is indicated. Where the site of bleeding is known a segmental resection is appropriate.

OBSTRUCTION

Natural history

Obstruction is usually incomplete and normally a feature of chronic disease. It is however the main reason for presentation in 10% of patients with complicated diverticular disease.

Acute obstruction may be due to colonic oedema or fibrosis and the inflammatory phlegmon may involve the small bowel in acute diverticulitis. Both small and large bowel obstruction may also be the result of adhesions secondary to previous extracolonic inflammation.

Clinical presentation

See Chapter 34.

Careful clinical assessment is required to differentiate between paralytic ileus secondary to peritonitis and mechanical obstruction.

Investigations

- Check blood for fluid and electrolyte status.
- Plain abdominal radiographs may show colonic oedema with stricturing and proximal dilatation. Isolated small bowel obstruction may be a feature in adhesional obstruction.
- Contrast studies or colonoscopy may be indicated to assess the calibre and length of a stricture and to exclude malignant change.

Management

See Chapter 34.

Conservative treatment

Often the obstruction is partial and settles with conservative management including bowel rest, intravenous antibiotics (as for acute diverticulitis) and parenteral fluids.

Surgery

- Most patients (87%) presenting acutely with obstruction will require surgery.
- Segmental resection with primary anastomosis is preferred providing the bowel wall is healthy and the bowel can be either preoperatively prepared or cleared by intraoperative colonic lavage. Alternatively exteriorisation of the proximal colon with closure of the distal limb (Hartmann's procedure) may be indicated.

Endoscopic treatment

- Patients unfit for surgery may be treated by endoluminal stent which is inserted by a combined endoscopic and radiological approach.
- This has also been advocated as a means of decompressing the bowel prior to elective surgery.

Further reading

1   Bailey I, Tate JJT. Acute conditions of the small bowel and appendix. In: Paterson-Brown S, ed. *A companion to specialist surgical practice: emergency surgery and critical care*. London: WB Saunders, 1997: 187–212.
2   Campbell KL, Munro A. Acute conditions of the large intestine. In: Paterson-Brown S, ed. *A companion to specialist surgical practice: emergency surgery and critical care*. London: WB Saunders, 1997: 151–86.
3   Keighley MRB. Left-sided colonic diverticular disease. In: Keighley MRB, Williams NS, ed. *Surgery of the anus, rectum and colon*. London: WB Saunders, 1993: 1128–211.
4   Memon MA, Fitztgibbons RJ. The role of minimal access surgery in the acute abdomen. *Surg Clin N Am* 1997: 77(6): 1333–53.
5   Parks TG. Natural history of diverticular disease of the colon. *Clin Gastroenterol* 1975; **4**: 53–69.
6   Painter NS, Burkitt DP. Diverticular disease of the colon, a 20th century problem. *Clin Gastroenterol* 1975; **4**: 3–22.

39 Acute lower gastrointestinal haemorrhage: specific conditions

with contributions from John Moorehead, Paul Neilly

Introduction

The causes of acute lower gastrointestinal haemorrhage are discussed in Chapter 6. Please see Table 6.1 in that chapter. Some of the more common causes will be discussed.

MECKEL'S DIVERTICULUM

Clinical presentation

This occurs in 1–3% of the population, is normally within 100 cm of the ileocaecal valve and contains oxyntic mucosa in 45%. Bleeding usually occurs in young children (mean age 5 years) and is typically recurrent, presenting as a mixture of melaena and dark red rectal bleeding. Bleeding is usually from ulcers in nearby intestinal mucosa. Adults often present with abdominal pain related to ulceration or other complications such as Meckel's diverticulitis, intussusception or perforation.

Management

- The diagnosis is made by $^{99}Tc^{m}$-pertechnetate scanning (positive in 75%) or selective mesenteric angiography.
- Surgical resection is required to excise both the diverticulum and the site of ulceration.

ANGIODYSPLASIA

Clinical presentation

Although these lesions may be found in any part of gastrointestinal tract, 80% affect the terminal ileum or proximal colon. They are more common in elderly patients (25%) and are responsible for 30–40% of lower gastrointestinal bleeds. The bleeding may be chronic and occult with iron deficiency anaemia but most (85%) present as acute painless overt haemorrhage which is often recurrent.

Management

- The lesions are seen at colonoscopy as elevated patches composed of prominent vessels that bleed on contact.
- Diathermy (preferably bipolar), heater probe and Nd-YAG laser coagulation are all recognised methods of endoscopic treatment.
- Mesenteric angiography can identify lesions and can be used therapeutically using vasopressin.
- Surgical resection is required for recurrent bleeding or extensive patches of angiodysplasia that cannot be otherwise treated.

DIVERTICULOSIS

Clinical presentation

This is the commonest cause of colonic haemorrhage and in 60% of these individuals the bleeding arises from the ascending or transverse colon. Bleeding is usually major and continuous but rarely causes hypovolaemic shock. In contrast the bleeding associated with angiodysplasia is often intermittent. Although the bleeding stops within 24 h of presentation in most patients (55%) with diverticular disease 25% of these patients will rebleed. Most patients are elderly (>70 years) with associated co-morbidity precluding extensive investigation or surgical management. Hypertension is a common association and may account for the spontaneous resolution occurring with relative hypotension following a major bleed.

233

Management

- If patients are otherwise fit, investigations and management should follow the previously described pattern for lower gastrointestinal haemorrhage (Chapter 6, Figure 6.1).
- Bleeding usually arises from the right colon (60%) and confirmed persistent bleeding from this site requires a right hemicolectomy.
- If the source of bleeding is uncertain an abdominal colectomy with ileorectal anastomosis is required.

HAEMORRHOIDS

Clinical presentation

Haemorrhoids classically present with bright red bleeding which either drips from the anus or coats the stool on defaecation. In the absence of thrombosis and oedema haemorrhoids are usually painless. It is rare for haemorrhoids to cause anaemia or hypovolaemia but this may be associated with portal hypertension.

Management

- Conservative management includes a high fibre diet $\pm$ bulking agents to reduce the pressure at the anorectal junction.
- Ointments, suppositories and other topical preparations have no proven role in the management of painless haemorrhoids.
- Small bleeding haemorrhoids (grade 1 and 2) can be treated by injection sclerotherapy or infrared coagulation.
- Larger internal haemorrhoids (grade 2 and 3) are best managed by rubber band ligation or haemorrhoidectomy.
- Grade 4 lesions usually require a formal haemorrhoidectomy.

CARCINOMA

Clinical presentation

Carcinomas in the small bowel or right colon rarely present with overt rectal bleeding. Carcinoma of the colon accounts for 5–10% of overt rectal bleeding with the lesion either in the left hemicolon or rectum. Right-sided colonic lesions usually present with occult bleeding and iron deficiency anaemia. Malignant invasion of blood vessels may however give massive rectal bleeding from any site.

Management

- Curative management of malignant small bowel and colorectal tumours requires surgical resection.
- Metachronous tumours occur in 3% of colorectal cancer cases. This justifies surveillance colonoscopy particularly in patients where there is synchronous polypoid change in the remaining colon. The average lag period between polyp formation and malignant change is 10 years. Surveillance procedures every 3-5 years are therefore sufficient.

POLYPS

Clinical presentation

Colonic polyps rarely cause symptoms unless they are large (>2 cm) or multiple (>20). Rectal bleeding is the most common feature with adenomatous polyps (44%) but other causes for bleeding such as haemorrhoids often co-exist. Large villous adenomas usually present with diarrhoea and large quantities of bloody mucus. Unless directly visualised it should never be assumed that the sole cause of bleeding in patients with rectal polyps are the polyps themselves.

Management

- Colonoscopy or contrast radiology is required to exclude tumours or inflammation proximal to the rectum.
- All polyps should ideally be removed and most polyps (95%) proximal to the rectum can be excised endoscopically.
- Large sessile polyps, depending on the degree of dysplasia, may be removed piecemeal using repeated procedures over several months.
- Multiple or large sessile polyps with moderate/severe dysplasia usually require primary surgical resection.
- Malignant polyps may be treated endoscopically provided the stalk is narrow and free of tumour. Histological evidence however of lymphatic or vascular invasion may justify surgical resection following polypectomy. In this situation early endoscopy

may be required to identify the polypectomy site and tattoo it with Indian ink to assist with subsequent surgical resection.

INFLAMMATORY BOWEL DISEASE

Clinical presentation

Rectal bleeding is a feature in 60% of patients with ulcerative colitis and Crohn's colitis. The severity of bleeding and anaemia correlates with disease activity. Proctitis usually presents as fresh red bleeding whereas more proximal disease gives dark red blood mixed with the stool. Inflammatory bowel disease rarely results in major haemorrhage.

Management

- It is important to differentiate idiopathic inflammatory bowel disease from infective enterocolitis that usually requires microscopic examination and stool culture.
- Biopsy is also essential, as negative bacteriological assessment does not necessarily exclude an infective cause.
- Most patients can be managed medically (see Section III: Chapters 34 and 36) but approximately 2% of patients with ulcerative colitis and 1% with Crohn's colitis require urgent surgery for haemorrhage.

Further reading

1 Beck DE. Hemorrhoidal disease. In: Beck DE, Wexner SD, eds. *Fundamentals of anorectal surgery*. London: WB Saunders, 1998: 237–53.
2 Carter DC. Non-neoplastic structural disease of the colon. In: Shearman DJC, Finlayson NDC, Camilleri M, Carter DC, eds. *Diseases of the gastrointestinal tract and liver*. London: Churchill Livingstone, 1997: 1379–98.
3 Demarkles MP, Murphy JR. Acute lower gastrointestinal bleeding. *Med Clin N Am* 1993;**73**:1085–100.
4 Forbes A (ed). *Clinicians' guide to inflammatory bowel disease*. London: Chapman & Hall, 1997.
5 Foutch PG. Angiodysplasia of the gastrointestinal tract. *Am J Gastroenterol* 1993;**88**(6):807–18.
6 Keighley MRB. Bleeding from the colon and rectum. In: Keighley MRB, Williams NS, eds. *Surgery of the anus, rectum and colon*. London: WB Saunders, 1993: 1926–70.
7 Lewis BS. Small intestinal bleeding. *Gastroenterol Clin N Am* 1994;**23**:67–91.
8 Phillips RKS ed. *A companion to specialist surgical practice: colorectal surgery*. London: WB Saunders, 1998.
9 Vernava AM III, Moore BA, Longo WE, Johnson FE. Lower gastrointestinal bleeding. *D Colon Rectum* 1997;**40**(7):846–58.

Index

Page numbers in **bold** type refer to figures, and those in *italics*, to tables